I0199290

"I believe we will reach a point where we won't segregate our mentally ill and mentally retarded. We will recognize they are us."

—Dr. Lloyd Elam

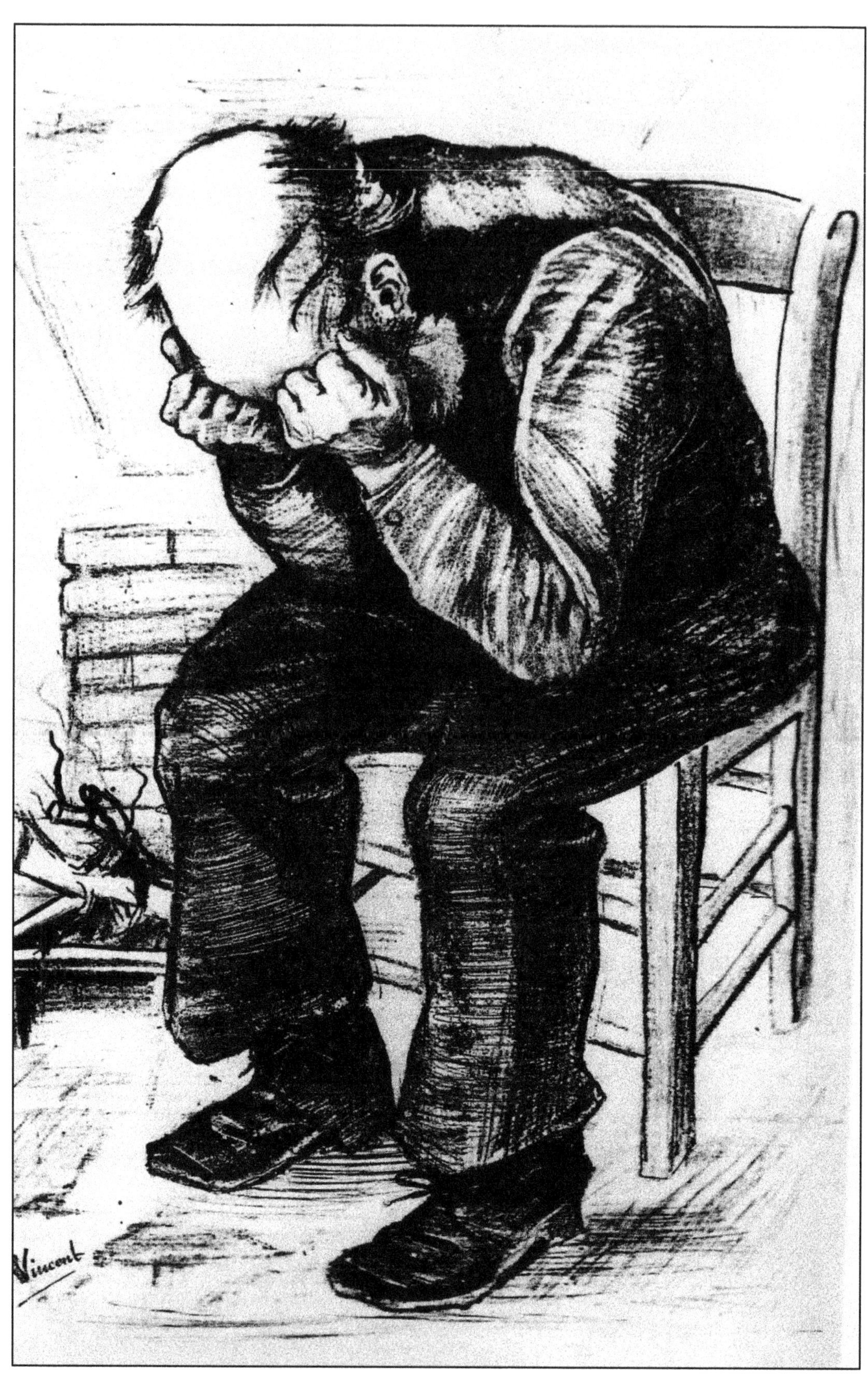

Van Gogh's *At Eternity's Gate*, a lithograph from 1882

THEY ARE US

(What People with Mental Illness Have Taught Me)

Part One —History and Observations
Part Two —Stories about Mental Illness
Part Three —Words to Politicians and Others

By

George Spain, MSSW

Ideas into Books: Westview®
Kingston Springs, Tennessee

Ideas into Books®
W E S T V I E W
P.O. Box 605
Kingston Springs, TN 37082
www.publishedbywestview.com

The second section of this book is a work of fiction. Names, characters, places and incidents either are products of the author's imagination or are used fictitiously. Any resemblance to actual events or locales or persons, living or dead, is entirely coincidental.

ISBN 978-1-62880-158-3

First edition, November 2018

Printed in the United States of America on acid free paper.

PROLOGUE

The time was when insanity in all forms and degrees, regardless of causes that may have preceded, was attributed to satanic agency. The unfortunate individual was considered a demoniac, possessed of devils who drove him at will from place to place, and into all excess of violence and insanity. Such cases as these, in the opinion of that age, could only be managed by supernatural means, such as charms, incantations, or miraculous interpositions.... We only affirm that the frequent instances of mental derangement which occur in our day are of a very different character, and require different treatment. The former being a supernatural affection could not be counteracted and controlled by a supernatural power of greater force. The latter being the result of some irregularity in the physical organs, may of course be restored, by restoring the original course of these organs.... It is a fact that insanity is a disease subject to ordinary treatment.

—John D. Kelley, M.D.
Superintendent, Lunatic Asylum of Tennessee
1843 Report to the Tennessee Legislature

DEDICATION

To

All Who Have a Mental Illness and Their Families

and

Dorothea Lynde Dix
W. P. Jones, M.D.
and always, Jackie

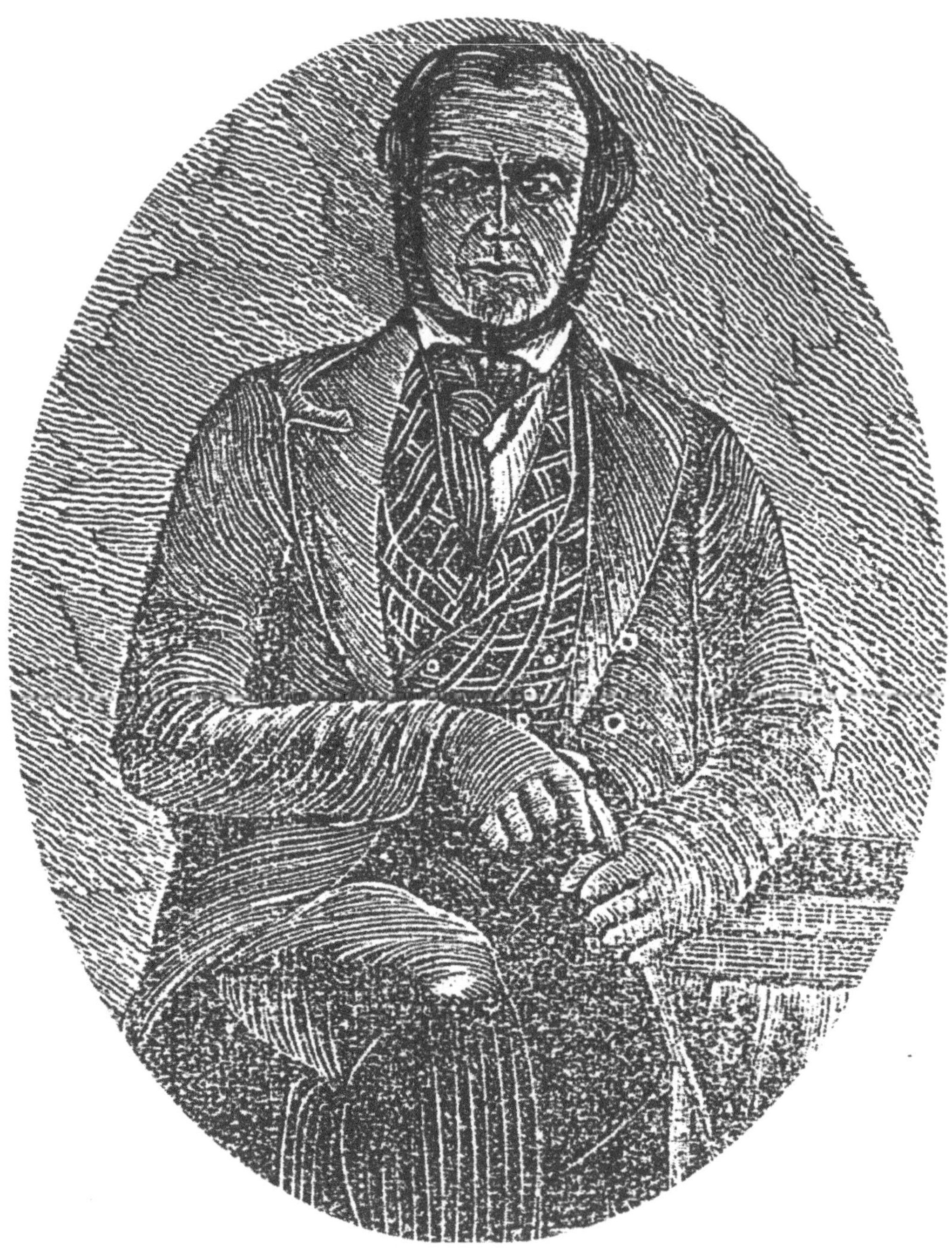

Green Grimes

"Gentlemen and ladies in high station.
Will you look down upon the insane and idiot,
With contempt? You and your great relations
Might all become maniacs and idiot,
Will you turn to them a deaf ear,
Or will you raise your voice for them in prayer,
That God may restore their minds and bless you every year,
And lead them from the dangerous snare?
They are of the same dust and fellow being,
Your conduct is marked down
By the eyes of Him who is always seeing,
He expects you in your duty to be found.
If you should mistreat them and show disrespect,
Slim would be your chance for heaven;
Therefore you had better them protect,
That you and them may be pure leaven,
Thus you may wear fine laurels,
And meet them in peace beyond Jordan's stormy banks,
Where never enter jars or quarrels;
Where you would win crowns, golden harps and thanks."

—Green Grimes
Admitted to Lunatic Asylum of Tennessee in 1842.

A SECRET WORTH KNOWING

A TREATISE

ON THE

MOST IMPORTANT SUBJECT IN THE WORLD:

SIMPLY TO SAY,

INSANITY,

THE ONLY WORK OF THE KIND IN THE UNITED STATES, OR, PERHAPS, IN THE KNOWN WORLD, FOUNDED ON GENERAL OBSERVATION AND TRUTH.

There are other Medical books which treat on Insanity, but comparatively few to the population, and none written by an Insane man. This contains a short History of the Author's case—giving the General Causes which produced the Disease on him individually, Manner of Treatment and Termination. Giving the only Treatment by which a Cure may be effected, the Manner of Detecting the Disease, and the Duties of Sane Parents towards the Insane offspring of their bodies; with some general remarks upon Idiotism, the Jurisprudence of Insanity, Suicide, &c.

BY G[reen]. GRIMES,

AN INMATE OF THE LUNATIC ASYLUM OF TENNESSEE.

NASHVILLE, TENN.

1846.

APPRECIATION

For many years the following have guided and supported me in my writing: Carolyn Wilson, Maxine and Harry Rose, Babs and Deems Brooks, Bob Scruggs, Tommy Burton, Sandy Zeigler and the Williamson County Writers Critique Group—thank you all.

And special thanks to my long time editors, Gayle and Jerry Henderson—they have smoothed down the rough places and filled in the holes I had not seen.

As always a hurrah to that best of publishers, Mary Catharine Nelson.

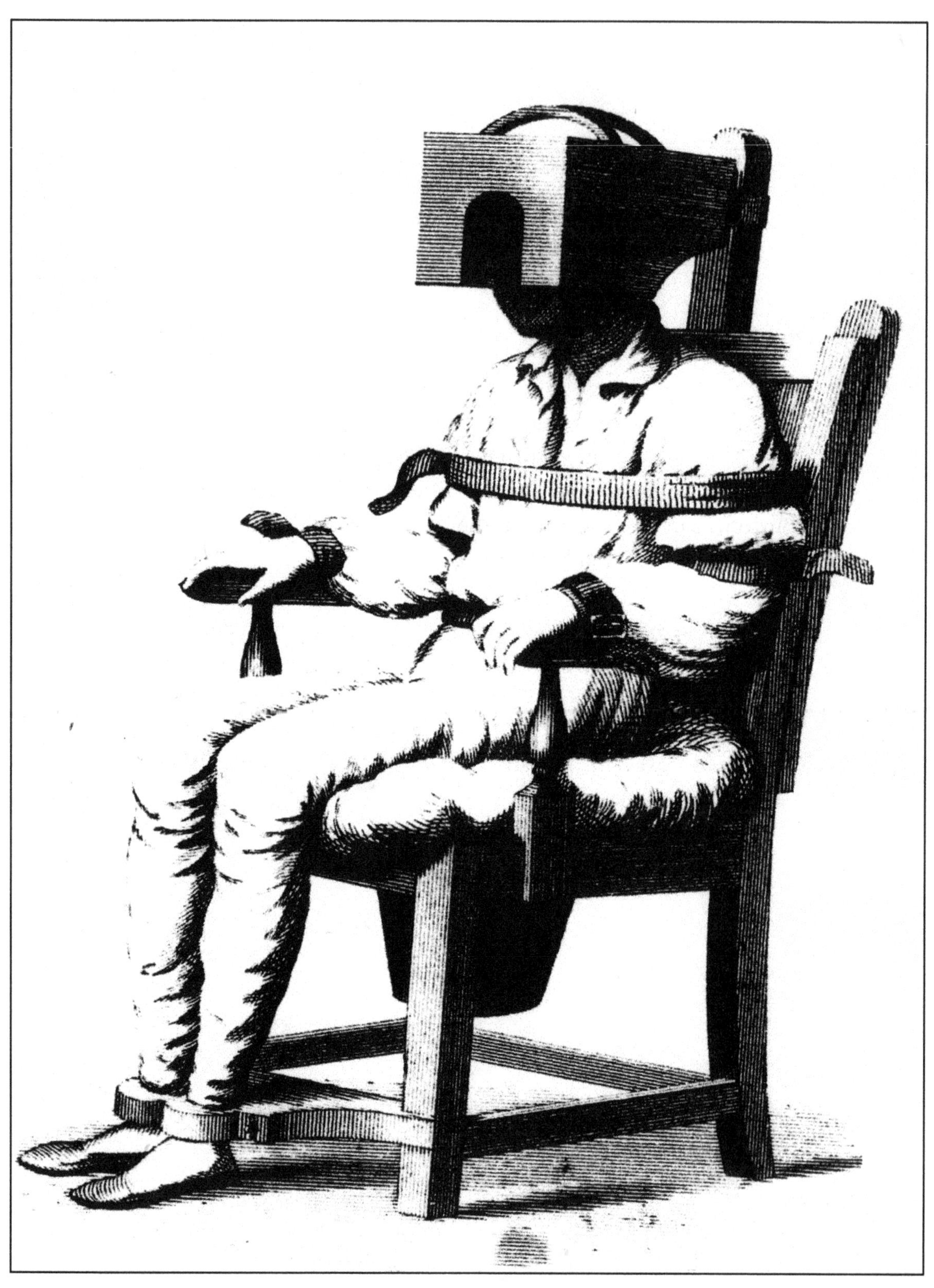

Benjamin Rush's "Tranquillizer" from the *Philadelphia Medical Museum* (1911)

"In the distant future I see open fields for far more important researches. Psychology will be based on a new foundation, that of the necessary acquirement of each mental power and capacity by gradation. Light will be thrown on the origin of man and his history."

Charles Darwin
On the Origin of the Species
1859

"...We have been inclined to take the opposite view, that in mental life nothing which has once been formed can perish—that everything is somehow preserved and that in suitable circumstances...it can once more be brought to light...an entity, that is to say, in which nothing has once come into existence will have passed away and all the earlier phases of development continue to exist alongside the latest one."

Sigmund Freud
Civilization and Its Discontents
1929

"There ain't nobody that don't sometime in life get hung up in a brier patch and don't know which way to turn to get out."

A Tennessee Country Woman

"If a man does not keep pace with his companions, perhaps it is because he hears a different drummer. Let him step to the music he hears.... Could a greater miracle take place than for us to look through each other's eyes for an instant."

Henry David Thoreau
Walden

"With all our stupidities and failures, there is something in most of us that keeps trying to do better, and sometimes it happens; sometimes, beyond ourselves, we even try to make things better for others—and sometimes we do."

George Spain

TABLE OF CONTENTS

PART ONE

HISTORY AND OBSERVATIONS

I'm not a medical doctor, a molecular biologist, not even a trained historian. But in the Tennessee State Archives I found, read and copied almost everything on the early conditions and treatment of people with mental illness: some were chained and locked in homes, some lived in caves and poorhouses, many wandered alone, and others, as now, were in jails.

This is a story about what was, is, and one day might be.

I'd guess you are probably like me. Either someone in your family, yourself or a friend has, or has had, some form of mental illness or severe emotional problem. Mental illnesses are among the most common diseases that afflict humans. Among the most severe are: schizophrenia which affects one percent of us; manic-depression (bipolar) another one percent; major depression, ten to twenty percent; and Alzheimer's, fifteen percent of those over sixty-five years of age. Added to those comes the heart breaker—suicide—which leaves many lingering questions never to be answered and condemnations and guilt that may punish their surviving loved ones until they die. Ten percent of people with schizophrenia and ten percent of those with severe depression die by suicide. David Guth, my friend and co-founder of Centerstone Community Mental Health Centers and now its Chief Executive Officer, added that, "Presently, ten percent of patients with anxiety disorders result in suicide if left untreated, and substance abuse is now our single largest health crisis."

To whet your interest for what's coming, let me begin with a personal experience. As said, there are lots of things I am not but there once came a day in the mid-1970s when I was Jesus for just a little while. It was during the fuel crisis and the government was pushing the country to carpool. Being Director of the Columbia Area Mental Health Center in Columbia, Tennessee, I thought I should set an example for our employees. Every morning I drove to Franklin in my Volkswagen van and picked up three colleagues: C.C., our chief psychologist who could be tough as a ten-penny nail, and two young caseworkers.

On US Highway 31, between Franklin and Columbia, was an almost-nonexistent hamlet called Thompsons Station. It was made up of a crossroad; a store; an antebellum house; an empty, crumbling schoolhouse; farmland, and all the sky above the fields and rolling hills. On this particular morning, a truck was parked on the far side of the road a hundred yards from the store. As we passed I saw a man lying in the gravel beside the truck. I turned the van around at the store and went back. As the tires crunched in the gravel, I stopped fifty feet away from the truck and told C.C. to take the wheel. “I'll go and see what's wrong.” I smiled and said, “But if he jumps up and is about to attack me, get me in the van or run over him.”

I got out and walked cautiously toward the man who was stretched out on his back still as death. As I walked toward him I began to talk in my kindest, softest mental-health voice, “Hey, fellow...are you okay?” No answer. No movement. Forty feet away...a little louder, “Hey there!” Nothing. Thirty feet..."Are you okay?” Twenty feet and loudly this time, “SIT UP IF YOU CAN OR SAY SOMETHING.” Not a twitch or sound. My leg muscles were ready to run. Ten feet...five...a gaunt, gray-pallored man lay there; not of much size, he was wearing loose fitting, filthy, once-white-paint-splattered bib overalls and one brogan. Greasy, uncombed hair hung down to his shoulders. He stank to high heaven from pee and whiskey. I stood at his feet and with the toe of my shoe nudged the sole of his brogan, when...*O MY LORD!*

His eyes flicked open. He smiled, sat up, and leaning against the truck, looked straight up into my eyes and said, “Lord Jesus, you've come.”

My chest pounding I stepped back, my eyes wide and fixed, my feet prepared to jump. *What'n hell...Well, I'll be damned! He's drunk...I'll be damned.* As either Charles Darwin or Mark Twain said, “In certain trying circumstances, urgent circumstances, desperate circumstances, profanity furnishes a relief denied even to prayer.” Now I think about it that sounds more like Twain than Darwin, don't you think?

If you have a Master's degree in psychiatric social work and have worked in the Department of Psychiatry at Vanderbilt, plus having been schooled for sixteen years at David Lipscomb, a Church of Christ school, where you had Bible class an hour and a half a day, coupled with going to church and Sunday school since you were in diapers, how do you respond to someone who has just called you “Jesus”? I reached down and said, “Take my hand and come with me.” He took my hand and I lifted him up. We put him in the van and drove to Maury Regional Hospital. He was having alcoholic hallucinations. I took him into the emergency room and after a bit, left...and also left Jesus with him.

This story is just one of many from my life experiences with people who have been called lunatics, crazy, insane, mad, demon-possessed, mentally ill, or have had a genetic brain disease. When you have come to the end of this book I hope you will see that it is really a story about you and me. As my friend, Dr. Lloyd Elam, wrote in 1978, "I believe we will reach a point where we won't segregate our mentally ill and mentally retarded. We will recognize they are us." We've come a long way, yet with all our advanced knowledge and sophistication, there remains the voice of the Pharisee who prays, "God, I thank Thee that I am not as other men." So we continue to fear mental illnesses, such as schizophrenia and bipolar disorder, as we do cancer, and most tend to be uncomfortable around those who have them. Nor have we yet, with all our vaunted research, found a way to prevent them.

"We will carry each other around in our hearts forever." So said Wind Bird, a young Cherokee girl from East Tennessee, those exact words to me in 1966 as she was leaving my office in the Vanderbilt Department of Psychiatry for the last time. She stood there in the doorway. Her eyes and short-cropped hair were coal-black. Her skin was like my grandfather's, olive-dark, much darker than my whiteness. I had been her therapist for three years. She was returning to her home in the foothills of the Smokies.

To Wind Bird and all who have been a part of my more than fifty years in mental health: Thank you and your families for teaching me things I would have never known but for your words and your perseverance to make things better for yourselves and the rest of us.

Who are we? How did we get here? How were we formed? What is it about our brains and how they work? Where do we go from here? These questions have tangled in my head as far back as I have known to ask them. Jackie, my wife, once asked me, with a tad of frustration in her voice, "Don't you ever give your brain a rest?"

Sitting comfortably in the recliner she had given me the previous Christmas, I stopped doodling architectural drawings for a low energy house and thought for a moment...then another...and said, "Well...huh...I guess I can't; it just keeps going on and on all the time."

So the questions and answers at the heart of this book come to me. There are probably some discrepancies here, some purposeful for confidentiality, others because of lapses in memory, some because of personal judgment.

From 1957 to 2007 I worked as a psychiatric social worker, mental health therapist, administrator, and advocate for the mentally ill in Tennessee. Now, at eighty-one, as I look back over my life I see teachers everywhere and of every sort: family members, friends and colleagues. Those of a different sex, age, and nationality from myself. Some who taught me were mentally ill whom I met in jails and prisons and hospitals, two on the roadside, one under a bridge; most living alone, some were estranged from their families. There were those of every color, race, religion. Some rich enough to 'barbecue a white elephant'; others were 'poor as church mice'. There were legislators, judges, professors, and corporate leaders, a few killers, drug dealers, bank robbers and a demolition expert for the Ku Klux Klan, but most were hard-working, church-going, middle-class folks with their scattering of problems.

They taught me truths that have never left me. No one comes into this world perfect, everyone arrives here with a built-in weakness: some little, some big, some are recognizable from a first glance, other symptoms are evidenced gradually. In like manner, I found that most of those I came to really know had a piece of goodness inside, what I came to call, 'a piece of gold'.

Though I've heard and seen a whole bunch of misery, I still believe Jesus is our best example, even while there are lots of things in the Bible that are cruel—too cruel—which I despise and will never accept as coming from a "loving God". Except for those few people who seem to be cruel to the bone, I want to believe that even they, like the rest of us, need compassion in their lives, especially when they come to their end.

One of my favorite writers, Mark Twain, put it this way, "There's a good spot tucked away somewhere in everybody. You'll be a long time finding it sometimes."

A hero of mine states it perfectly. Winston Churchill said, "Human beings are endowed with infinitely varying qualities and dispositions, and each one is different from the other. We cannot make them all the same. It would be a pretty dull world if we did."

Hearing Twain and Churchill speak leads me to restate what I have written above. But, as I've delved into writing this book, I've rethought my words and decided to add: There are exceptions to everybody having 'a piece of gold'. Now and then, an exception comes along. a cruel psychopath, someone filled with hate almost from birth, who abuses, tortures and kills animals and humans without any apparent remorse. Thank God that this malady is rare. So the question comes, if you believe in God ask yourself why does He allow these beings to exist among us. Putting it off on Satan or saying it is beyond our knowing is not good enough for me. We need to delve more deeply and comprehensively for answers. I believe they are hiding in plain sight and are just waiting to be discovered by the next student psychiatrist leader...could it be you?

Yes, some of the people I worked with acted strange, some scary, a few dangerous but not one was 'evil', not even the psychopath. And not one was as they were because of a supernatural being. As Dr. Elam said, "... They are us."

Some believe God created man and "the heavens and the earth", others believe it all began with a 'big bang', still others believe in evolution. Many believe all three and, of course, there are those who don't really have an opinion. But I believe how we believe leads to how we see one another, especially our differences in behavior.

"That there is much suffering in the world no one disputes. Some have attempted to explain this in reference to man by imagining that it serves for his moral improvement. But the number of men in the world is as nothing compared with that of all other sentient beings, and these often suffer greatly without any moral improvement. A being so powerful as a God who could create the universe, is to our finite minds omnipotent and omniscient, and it revolts our understanding to suppose that his benevolence is not unbounded, for what advantage can there be in the sufferings of millions of the lower animals throughout almost limitless time? This very old argument from the existence of suffering against the existence of an intelligent first cause seems to me a strong one; whereas...the presence of much suffering agrees well with the view that all organic beings have been developed through variation and natural selection."

Charles Darwin
Charles Darwin's Autobiography

A HISTORY OF MENTAL ILLNESS

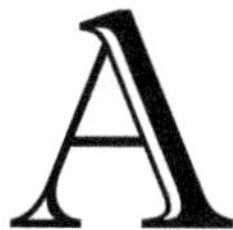s early as 1000 B.C., the Old Testament tells of David's fleeing from Saul's anger. He fled to Gath and was brought before King Achish where,

> *He changed his behavior before them, and he feigned himself mad in their hands, and he scrabbled on the doors of the gate, and let his spittle fall down upon his beard. Then said Achish unto his servants, 'Lo, ye see the man is mad wherefore have ye then brought him to me? Have I need of mad men, that ye have brought this fellow to play the mad man in my presence? Shall this fellow come into my house?'*
>
> First Samuel 21:10-15

In John 10:20 of the New Testament, it also says about Jesus, *And many of them said, He hath a devil, and is mad, why hear ye him?* And what did He do? He cast a demon out of a man into a herd of hogs who ran off a cliff into the sea and drowned themselves—what the FDA would judge to be 'possessed pork'.

Next in history come the witches! Since the Dark Ages, man has been concerned over the power of witches. As time progressed, it seems that more people incanted and chanted and did scary things. Many, mostly women, were accused of witchcraft. Thousands upon thousands were hanged or burned, nine hundred in the city of Bamberg, Germany alone.

And then came 1692 in Salem, Massachusetts. Arthur Miller's play, *The Crucible*, describes some of those young, genteel, religious girls (Elizabeth Parris, Abigail Williams, Mercy Lewis, Ann Putnam, and others) as they had convulsive fits, swooning and choking spells, loss of appetite, saw strange animals, saw a man in black, and accused neighbors of witchcraft. Reverend John Hale, the respected pastor of Salem, described them: "Their arms, necks, and backs were turned this way and that way, and returned back again so as it was impossible to do of themselves, and beyond the power of any epileptic fits, or natural disease to effect." Dr. William Griggs provided the diagnosis of the day. "The evil hand is upon them." Before the pandemonium was over, nineteen were hung, one pressed to death, and one hundred imprisoned and impoverished.

In the late 1950s I saw the same behavior, which Reverend Hale had described, on the back ward of the Davidson County Hospital. As I opened the heavy thick door to the male ward, I could hear birdcall chatterings and insect clickings like those in the Amazon jungle. Opening the door wider I could see long benches built against each wall, occupied by men twisting, jerking, some unmoving, statuesque, silent. I had entered a jungle.

Those accused of "familiarity with the devil" were sometimes ill-mannered troublemakers among their neighbors. For witchcraft accusations to be filed, certain elements were needed: a belief in witchcraft, harms falling upon the community, crop failures, epidemics, controversies, plagues, comets, and storms in the heavens. Can you imagine the fear and uncertainty that was created? What was causing these calamities? How could they be controlled? Who was to blame? Who better to accuse than the Devil and his followers.

Though he did not prevent the hangings, a Boston cloth merchant spoke out against Cotton Mather and other church leaders caught up in the Salem frenzy:

"That there are witches is not in doubt, the Scriptures else were in vain which assigns their punishment to be by death. But what this witchcraft is, or wherein it does consist, seems to be the whole difficulty."

Robert Calef
Salem
1700

Also, there were some Salem participants in the accusations and final judgments who later lamented their behavior:

> "Great hardships were brought upon innocent persons, and [we fear] guilt incurred, which we have all cause to bewail."
>
> Reverend Cotton Mather

> "As I was a chief instrument of accusing Goodwife Nurse and her two sisters, I desire to lie in the dust, and to be humbled for it." [Rebecca Nurse was hanged in July 1692.]
>
> Ann Putnam

Here in Tennessee in the early 1800s, arguably, we had the most famous witch in our country's history: the Bell Witch. Come with me for a moment to Adams, a small farming village north of Nashville on the Tennessee/Kentucky border. On the backside of the Bell farm runs the Red River, which winds close to my grandparents' farm in Schochoh, Kentucky. When I was a little boy I spent weeks during the summers with them. At night, after supper, I would sit with them on the front porch and listen to their stories. My favorite, which scared the dickens out of me and never left, was about the Bell Witch.

A half mile or so from the only store in Adams is the neat, almost quarter-of-an-acre Bellwood cemetery surrounded by a low white wall. The tombstones are regularly spaced around a tall white monument. Standing in the cemetery on a late, gray, fall day in 1994, looking east across a large, plowed, dry-stubble corn field, I saw a distant line of bare trees. Wind rustled the dry corn leaves. Surrounding me were the dead descendants of John Bell Sr., one of the first settlers in middle Tennessee. His house once stood not far out in the field. His and his wife's bones are buried somewhere nearby, but no one has found their graves. I love to bring my grandchildren here for picnics.

The *Spirit*, as the Bell family came to call it, has come down to us as the *Bell Witch*. It first appeared in 1817 as a strange dog standing in a cornfield. It appeared again as a large bird, a young girl swinging on a tree limb, and then it came into the Bell home.

It quoted scriptures; sang; yanked the hair of Betsy, the Bells' daughter; knocked on doors and walls; dragged covers from beds; and said it would torment John Bell the rest of his life. The family prayed; their preacher, Reverend James Gunn, prayed; and the community prayed. John Bell choked, his face twitched and soon he died on December 20, 1820. A few months later whatever the Spirit was left and never returned.

According to John Bell's grandson, Charles Bailey Bell, the *Spirit* told Reverend Gunn that it was old Kate Batts' witch. Kate Batts, a married mother of six, lived two miles from the Bells. She was considered so odd that some in the community shunned her and suspected she practiced black magic. Many people began calling the *Spirit* Kate, and so it came to be known.[1]

What was it? A demon? A witch-woman? A *folie a deux*—a family's shared delusion—that spread through the community? Or was it a hoax by a top-notch storyteller? Can you guess which I believe?

So let me put the question to you in light of the beliefs of the twenty-first century. Was it possible that those accused of being witches were mentally ill? Maybe. Maybe not. Here are some things I have seen and heard about witches and demons.

From 1957 to 1958, I worked every Saturday at the old Davidson County Psychiatric Hospital in Bordeaux. One Saturday, two worried sisters of a genteel black lady came to give me a history about their sister's behavior. She, like her sisters, was gracious, but her thoughts and actions had become fixated on the fineness and fitness of her minister who she believed was 'hoodooing' her with locks of her hair and fingernail clippings. She began to say this to her sisters and upon hearing of this, the congregation became uneasy, so she was committed to the hospital.

In the summer of 1959 I worked as a student social worker at the long-departed Central State Psychiatric Hospital in Nashville. As part of a psychiatric team, I was asked to put together a history of a farmer who was convinced that witches lived on his farm. He had started painting white crosses on buildings and fence posts to contain them, but they continued to escape. So he took his bucket and brushes and began painting his neighbors' fence posts. That's where the trouble began. He was then committed to the hospital. He was a polite man but politeness did not control his delusions and hallucinations. When I left at the end of the summer he was still there.

When I tried to prevent a psychotic woman from leaving our ward in Maury Regional Hospital, she tried to scratch me because she thought I was Beelzebub. I remembered the man lying on the roadside having alcoholic hallucinations who thought I was Jesus. Neither the woman nor the man was influenced by the supernatural, both were mentally ill.

In the 1990s, a man came to our class at Woodmont Hills Church of Christ who professed to be a Godly preacher, a man highly respected by our church. He began to hold forth about a 'demon-possessed young girl'. He announced that he had "laid hands on her and cast out the demon."

My reaction was not a 'Hallelujah!' but, "*Well, I'll be damned.*"

You understand I said that in my head. I raised my hand and said, "Hold on! That's not right! You're wrong! She didn't have a demon in her. She was mentally ill." He stopped. The room was silent. And I'll give him credit, though he never backed down, he allowed some discussion. Three parents who were in the room at the time called me later to thank me on behalf of their mentally ill children. Shame on such stupidity coming from his mouth as though from God!

Holding such beliefs about the workings of God and the Devil, we might as well be down on our knees praying nightly, "From ghoulies and ghosties and long-legged beasties, good Lord, deliver us." It brings to mind Mark Twain's great theological observation that, "Man was made at the end of the week's work when God was tired." I would add that when He saw what a mess man was, God took a short nap and, waking up refreshed, He made woman.

It is important to add: The actual practice of witchcraft and the worship of Satan are not in and of themselves symptoms of mental illness. For most who have such beliefs, these are only manifestations of their differences in searching for understanding of themselves and others and of the unknown world beyond us.

The last legal execution for witchcraft in the British Isles was performed in 1722.

Of course, all those earlier centuries hadn't been filled with the Devil and evil. For many, maybe most, there was love and kindness. They believed God listened to them and that He sometimes spoke out loud to give hope and strength. This remains a belief of many today, but not all.

Let's end this depressing topic about witches with a one hundred and sixty-year-old poem written by Charles Upman in his 1867 book, *Salem Witches.*

Look out! Look out boys! Clear the tracks!
The Witches are here! They've all come back!
They hanged them high—No use! No use!
What cares a witch for a hangman's noose?
They buried them deeply, but they wouldn't lie still,
For cats and witches are hard to kill.

In 1751 Benjamin Franklin and the Quakers led the way in opening America's first hospital for the mentally ill in Pennsylvania. Franklin later said, "I do not remember any of my political maneuvers the success of which gave me at the time more pleasure."

I have often thought I should be a Quaker instead of a member of the Church of Christ. We, as do most churches, 'preach' peace but it's only the Quakers, Mennonites, and Amish who really 'practice' peace.

In 1792 Philippe Pinel, a French physician, unchained fifty 'maniacs' in a Paris hospital and originated the use of Moral Treatment.

Four years later, William Tuke, an English Quaker, started the Retreat in York, England, where religious principles, the Golden Rule, Christianity and basic kindness were to overcome the measureless violence of madness. Force and restraint were not to be used unless required by violent mania. Rather, there was to be a homelike setting with exercise, walks, conversation, and reading to shift dark thoughts into bright ones. Patients were encouraged to work, take trips, study art, poetry, music, and to have friends visit them.

Tuke opposed bleeding—a common practice of the day—recognizing that "medicine as yet possesses very inadequate means to relieve the most grievous of human diseases."

Philippe Pinel's approach and actions and Tuke's religious practices combined to form the principles of Moral Treatment which became the backbone of care that guided America through the mid- and late 1800s.

Asylums were to be located in an isolated area with pleasant grounds and clean, well-ventilated buildings, preferably with some farmland in order to provide opportunities for those patients who were able to work. The more disturbed patients were to be separated from the less disturbed.

Attendants were to be caring. The physician was to talk to the patient about his problems and interests with work; there was to be schooling, religious teaching, music, and carriage rides. Cold baths, wooden tranquilizer chairs, and leathern mittens were to be used as infrequently as possible. There was to be no harshness or cruelty. The mind was to be redirected and comforted.

A strong belief in curability was held in the mid-1800s. But it was not to be for those patients who suffered from severe mental conditions that were caused by illnesses in the brain.

In 1832, one hundred and forty-six Maury County Tennesseans petitioned the state legislature to set aside a "portion of the [new] Penitentiary house of our State for the lodging and comfortable keeping of the lunatics of our State. There is at present no provision for the proper maintenance of the unfortunate persons, some are confined in county jails, others are made inmates of poorhouses." It was recommended that there could be a "sort of hospital...allowing the lunatics to be under the care...of a regular physician." Lunatic was derived from the Latin word, Luna, which means moon. It was believed that the minds and behavior of people fluctuated with phases of the moon, as do the tides. So the words and beliefs about mental illness steadily evolved.[2]

About the same time that President Andrew Jackson used the army to uproot and remove the Cherokee from their ancient lands and send them across the Mississippi on the Trail of Tears, the Tennessee legislature approved ten thousand dollars to establish a hospital "out of brick or stone for at least two hundred patients." Eight years passed before the money was appropriated. It was built on the rise next to the railroad tracks a little ways off Eighth Avenue. It had only forty-three sleeping rooms. A small cupola crowned the top similar to the one on the new state penitentiary.

By 1840, Tennessee's population had grown to 800,000 and it was estimated that nine hundred to one thousand of its population were insane people. In the United States there were eighteen thousand.

Most of the insane were still in poorhouses and jails, some chained to or locked in their families' outhouses. We can't imagine the suffering of these people and their families.

Imagine standing in that cupola with Dr. John D. Kelly, the first superintendent and physician, whose annual salary was five hundred dollars. Beneath us is the brand new three-storied brick Lunatic Asylum of Tennessee where Dr. Kelly lives. If you turn and look across the railroad tracks down toward the Cumberland River, you can see the county jail.

It's March 28, there's still some bite in the air. We see a wagon coming from the direction of the jail. The wagon rolls up the drive and stops. The jailer climbs down and tells the two shackled men in the wagon bed to get out. We have come down from the cupola. Dr. Kelly treats them kindly. He asks the jailer to remove their shackles. After introducing himself he invites them inside as though they are guests and he is their host.

These men are from Lincoln County. They've been sitting in jail waiting for the hospital to open. Both are paupers. One is forty-five years old and married. He is maniacal. He's been this way for six years. He'll eventually get better and be discharged. The other is twenty-seven years old and single. He is also maniacal, possibly due to a head injury. He is incurable and will probably die in the asylum. As paupers each patient will cost the state two dollars and fifty cents a week.

They are examples of "maniacal" behavior. What brought about their ungovernable excitement and frenzy appears to differ. But there is nothing suggesting supernatural causes. They are examples of the increasing awareness that mental illness comes from inside ourselves, not from outside our own world, and not from God or the Devil.

Sixteen months after the asylum opened, Dr. Kelly writes in his first biannual report to the Legislature:

"Gentlemen...the objects of our peculiar regard, have with few exceptions, enjoyed most excellent health; and have been favored with every comfort which we could bestow. They appreciate our efforts for their intellectual and moral improvement have been crowned with success...in [this] benevolent and holy enterprise."

That's the way legal formality was once written.

"Thirty-one patients have been admitted, almost twice as many men as women. The majority are less than forty years old. Ten have been discharged, four died, one ran off. It has cost $5,490.35. The single highest item has been fresh meat: four hundred and thirty-six dollars. Food for two horses, a cow, and calf have cost $135.81. The paupers' clothing and replacement of things broken are $172.57; water casks and hauling water from the Cumberland River, $14.25; heating and cooking, $516.13. Revenue from the State and private patients, however, exceed the total cost."

Without reservation, John Kelly believes the medical and moral treatment being provided at the asylum will cure the disease of insanity if patients are brought for treatment early. He concluded his report urging education of the public "with a loud and earnest voice."

In June 1842, Green Grimes, a thirty-year-old man from Wayne County, is the thirty-first admission to the Lunatic Asylum. He is "melancholic [due to] pecuniary distress...in a freak of insanity and raving madness with a severe fit of epilepsy, he slashed his throat with a razor." He is a remarkable man. I discovered his two books in the state archives. Within three years of his admission he wrote *A Secret Worth Knowing* and *A Lily of the West*. Though the words are somewhat stiff and stylized they are filled with interesting poetry and details of his life and illness, and of other patients and treatments in the asylum. I may be wrong in my judgment, but when I read them there were still touches of depression, grandiosity and paranoia in his articulate and intelligent, historically important books.

What happened to him? I don't know. But on October 25, 1845, a male patient hanged himself with bed sheets from a window in the men's section.

Here's a typical day in the Nashville asylum in 1845: Rise at dawn; in the summer that's 4:30, in the winter 6:00. You dress, clean your room and the hall. Breakfast is two hours after rising, dinner at 12:30, supper at 6:00. There's plenty to eat: corn and wheat bread, soup, bacon, beef, vegetables, and molasses.

If you are a man you cut and carry wood, draw water, and work in the garden. If you are a woman you sew, knit, and wash dishes. Walking up and down the halls and in the yard, playing ball, cards or marbles, reading local newspapers, and maybe a book are the extent of your activities, except for Sunday. When a preacher is available, you are expected to dress your best and attend church services.

The day ends at 9:30.

These are the rules you live under:

1. You come with a thorough, written history of your illness.
2. You bring plenty of clothes.
3. Your snuff, tobacco, and money are held until you leave.
4. You have been told that this is an asylum and that you are here to be treated for mental derangement.
5. Your stay will depend upon the physician's judgment.
6. Your privileges depend upon your self-control and obeying the rules.
7. Men and women are separated all the time.
8. No "person of color" will be around you unless in the presence of the staff.
9. Your hands and face will be washed daily, your feet washed and hair combed and face shaved once a week. Clothes will be changed twice a week. Exercise daily.
10. No punishment is permitted except for cold baths. Attempts are made to avoid restraints, though, if absolutely necessary to

> control your violence, you may be put in a cold bath, straight waistcoat, or bound to a chair.

Dr. John McNairy takes over from Dr. Kelly in 1845. He details problems at the asylum in his report to the legislature. Rooms designed to hold twenty-one men now hold thirty-two with only two attendants. The cells below-ground where the violent are kept are "damp and gloomy and cannot be pure." A cistern is badly needed, as the wells do not provide enough water. Instead, water is being hauled from the river. In the winter the heating is so poor they have to gather as many patients as possible to huddle around a large fire.

Dr. McNairy tries to educate the legislature, "Insanity is a disease that can be cured, not the result of supernatural powers but from some irregularity in the physical organs, and, out of a population of 850,000 it is estimated that there are nine hundred to one thousand insane people who need help."

In 1847, our first hero arrives –

DOROTHEA LYNDE DIX

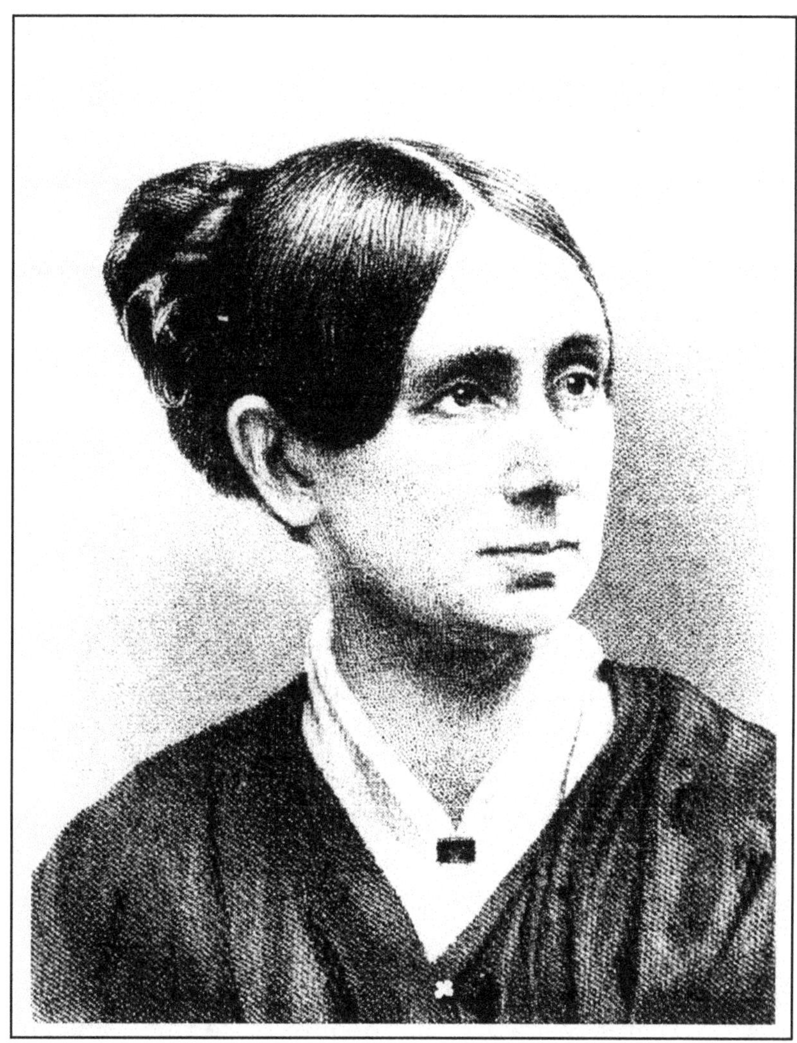

"In a world where there is so much to be done, I felt strongly impressed that there must be something for me to do."

—Dorothea Dix

What a woman! She arrives with a brain and tongue sharper than swords. She strides forth from New England into Tennessee to help the insane. You who are reading this think of heroes like Washington, Lincoln, Gandhi, Mandela, and King. They rose above the earth, but I'm telling you this rather frail, forty-six-year-old spinster and former schoolteacher was tough as they in mind and speech. She was one of those rare individuals who, now and then, stands, speaks out for those who have no voice, and makes a difference.

Between 1840, when she started her crusade across the nation, going into jails, poor farms and log cabins, until her death forty-five years later, she was a leader in bringing about the construction of thirty state hospitals for the insane, all the while educating politicians to the terrible conditions that existed and detailing recommendations for proper care and treatment.

She crisscrossed Tennessee. That October she wrote a "Memorial, Soliciting Enlarged and Improved Accommodations for the Insane of the State of Tennessee By the Establishment of a New Hospital"—a helluva of a long title!

Since women were not allowed to speak directly to the legislature, one legislator read it, had it copied and distributed to the entire esteemed body of gentlemen—none of whom were worthy of lacing her shoes.

She went right to the heart of the situation without mincing words. "The insane [are] in cells, dungeons, log cabins, bound with ropes, leather and chains, wandering alone and neglected, suffering in every county from the want of a suitable hospital." Then she went for the jugular, "How can Tennessee, which ranks number five in state populations, set the bad example of slighting the claims of her afflicted children? She is abundantly able to do this good work—she will do it, and she will do it now, freely, united, and well."

She told what she had experienced in her carriage travels to the horrific sights and smells of cells and hovels and poorhouses that contained insane human beings. Her descriptions are tough as railroad spikes. They are written by a heart and brain far beyond most people I have known.

Next she gave them a history lesson from Philippe Pinel. In the penitentiary she found "details too sickening and horrid to relate." And the Davidson County Poorhouse was "ill-repaired, cold, and cheerless with lunatics who suffer severely."

At the end of her Memorial she came to the crescendo of her exhortation with a long list of what they—the legislature—must do to rise to the challenge she had thrown at their feet. They must buy a farm with up to two hundred acres. It must have good water. It must have a brick building that will house two hundred lunatics and she adds, "Do not suffer wise economy to degenerate into meanness...Tennessee has been called the 'Mother of States'. Shall she not offer an example for the young states she has so largely and widely colonized."

On the last day of the legislative session, Senate Bill 131 passed for the new hospital. For a while they considered calling it the "Dix Hospital for the Insane of Tennessee". But state pride apparently overcame appreciation and it was named Tennessee Hospital For The Insane. In 1851 she sent the hospital a Bible and years later, three stereoscopes.

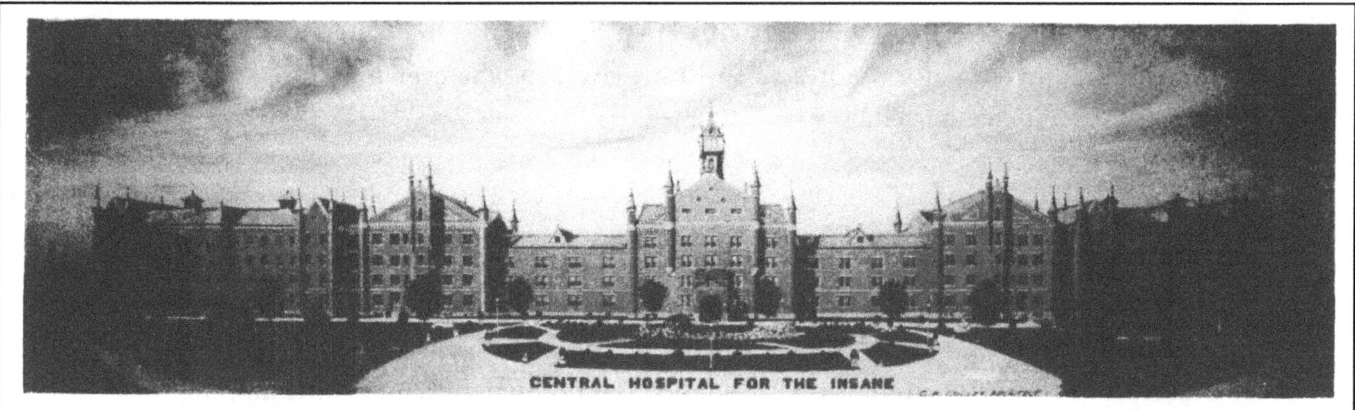

It was built pretty much as she wanted it. The new brick building was three hundred and twenty feet long, fifty feet wide and three to four stories high with one hundred and thirty-eight rooms. The castellated design was designated to have a tin roof and cast iron sashes over the windows. There was running water from a large reservoir and six hot furnaces, a chapel, parlor, library, private physician's apartment and a drug room. On the second floor was a "chastely furnished room for Miss Dix whenever it shall comport her convenience to visit the institution."

On April 19, 1852, sixty patients were moved from the old asylum to the new hospital and farm on Murfreesboro Pike, across from the present Metro Airport. The men were transported by train, the women by carriages.

Dorothea Lynde Dix shows us a life grandly lived yet most people don't even know her name. She is recognized in the Dedication of this book for her greatness to me and to the tens of thousands she helped.

From 1861 to 1865 she served as superintendent of Army nurses treating wounded Northern troops in the Civil War. After the war she continued to crusade for the mentally ill. Our country's greatest mental health advocate lived the last years of her life in a suite provided by the New Jersey legislature at the New Jersey State Hospital.

Heroes die just like the rest of us. On July 17, 1887, Dorothea Lynde Dix died and was buried in Mount Auburn Cemetery, Cambridge, Massachusetts. I am sorry that I have never visited her grave.

The following revelatory tribute to her was delivered to the Tennessee Legislature:

> She never married because of a sorrowful romance early in her life. She visited many U. S. states, and many of the first state hospitals in

this country were the direct results of her efforts. She visited England, Ireland, Scotland—the dungeons and leper houses of Rome, and Constantinople—for similar work and was received by Kings and by Prime Ministers. An audience with Pope Pius IX inspired the [Pope] to build a hospital for the insane in Rome. And in whatever presence, she never unsexed herself.

Back to the illness! What was causing it? Did it come from environmental influences, or hereditary causes? The lists given of causes stretch out: religious and political excitement, intemperance, masturbation, use of snuff, excessive study, disappointed love, and spirit rapping."

Many physicians who treated the mentally ill were turning away from supernatural causes. As Dr. McNairy stated, "The truth will probably be found in the assertion that insanity, like consumption and other afflictions, is the result of hereditary transmission, save where it can be explained by apparent physical disease." While an understanding of the illness was beginning to change, little was changing in treatment of "the violent patient who is confined in a chair [while] cold water is poured in a small stream on his head."

By 1855, two hundred and sixty-eight patients had been admitted. The building had grown to four hundred and nine feet long and one hundred feet wide, the bedrooms were eight by twelve feet. During this time there had been a severe outbreak of cholera but the hospital was not affected.

While Dr. William Cheatham, the new superintendent, was proud of the hospital, he was troubled that some physicians continued to believe that bleeding the insane, especially those with mania, was 'state of the art'. He emphatically stated, "Not so!" and proceeded to denounce this practice with examples: A man having four to five pounds of blood drawn from his body, resulted in his appearing bloodless though his "mind was still chaotic in the extreme."

In his 1859 report, he gives examples of moral changes in behavior that might be signs of insanity: a smooth tempered man who suddenly becomes irascible and insulting; a religious person who becomes profane and vulgar; and a "refined and educated woman...who becomes oblivious to the wickedest [of her] actions."

While ill health, religious excitement and family afflictions were considered major, hereditary predisposition was given as the leading cause of mental illness. Others given were: loss of loved ones or property, epilepsy, head injury, jealousy, immorality, pecuniary embarrassment, and exposure to heat.

There are eight pages in Dr. Cheatham's report to the legislature detailing the treatment of patients by the attendants: "Always with a pleasant smile; a cheerful, kind, and respectful manner; and with caring, sympathetic words." It would be wise for today's caregivers to heed the importance he attributed to basic kindness and good manners.

By 1860 the state's population had grown like kudzu to over one million and the new capitol building in Nashville had just been completed. The nation was rapidly moving toward the Civil War. Tennessee seceded from the Union the next year. The Lunatic Asylum was renamed the Tennessee State Hospital and was then controlled by the Medical Department of the University of Nashville.

And here's a funny side note: The old hospital in Nashville had been proposed as the Governor's mansion but after much discussion, it was voted down. What a shame!

Northern troops occupied Nashville and the hospital and its grounds in 1862. Andrew Johnson was appointed Military Governor. Poor Dr. Cheatham. His wife was sister to the confederate raider General John Morgan, so they were considered potential spies. The Federals replaced him with Dr. W. P. Jones, a northern sympathizer. The Cheathams moved quickly to Louisville where they remained until the end of the war.

In 1862, our second hero arrives –

DR. W. P. JONES

He was made like a muleskinner. In his way, he equaled Dorothea's heroics in Tennessee. He didn't have her fine ways and genteel words but he could bring hell down on you if you stood in his way of pursuing what he believed needed to be done. His well-honed knife blade tongue could whittle you down to the nubbins whether you were a Yankee or Rebel. He was smart, had a sense of humor, and was as bull-headed as an ox when fighting for the needs of the insane.

He ran the hospital from 1862 to 1869. In December 1864, the Union army defeated General Hood and the Confederate army in the hills a little south of Nashville. The war was almost over. Confusion abounded.

Dr. Jones's April 1865 Report

> "In the absence of the courts of the country, we have found it impossible to comply with the laws relative to the admittance of patients. And in lieu thereof...none have been refused who have furnished the right to admittance, by reasons of residence and insanity."

Three hundred and thirty-eight patients had been treated; one hundred and thirty-four were still in the hospital, including fifty-four soldiers. When the Union army had approached Nashville the officers of the Bank of Tennessee had escaped with the hospital's thirty thousand dollars, leaving it in financial straits.

Two divisions of Federal troops had been stationed on the hospital grounds in 1862. They had burned all the hospital's supply of wood, plus five miles of cedar fencing. Their horses had eaten sixty tons of hay. The troops stole one hundred thirty thousand bricks and all the livestock. They used the hospital for conferences. It was hell on earth. On top of everything else, a tornado blew part of the roof off the hospital and demolished the roofs of all the smokehouses, as well.

Only by giving the hospital's employees raises did they remain to care for the hundreds of patients. And our hero, Dr. W. P. Jones, rose to his greatness. Here is a list of some of the things he accomplished:

1. Before daylight, he, the farmhands and some patients went to the woods, chopped down trees, dragged them back and cut them into firewood.

2. He patched the roofs with tarpaulins and blankets.
3. During the winter of '64, "We—all hands—went merrily to work" cutting ice from ponds and filling two icehouses, which we sold for one thousand, five hundred and eighty-six dollars.
4. With his own money he bought clothes for the patients and charged them to their accounts.
5. With the stalwart farm foreman, George Richard, he oversaw the rebuilding of the cedar fencing the Yankees had burned and began planting and harvesting the fields.
6. Along with the gardener, Mr. Sharkey, he ran a flourishing greenhouse business that brought in two hundred and seventy dollars from plants and flowers.
7. He took care of his patients through it all; one hundred and thirty-one were discharged, and of these, one hundred and thirteen were recovered or improved.

Then he wrote, "The people of Tennessee have now decided that slavery and involuntary servitude, except as punishment for a crime...are forever abolished; and that the Legislature shall make no law recognizing the right of property in man."

Read that again because you can pass over its stylized wording without catching the grandeur of what he is saying. Let me rephrase what he was saying in plain English, "The days of black people being owned by white people are over."

Interspaced in the report are a few observations on the war and those who promoted it and participated. He was angry that the Federal army had stolen the hospital blind. But he had plenty left for preachers: "Most of the clergy of this country...very early became the leaders, aiders, and abettors of the rebellion. [While they preach] the duty of all men to be subject to the powers that be, they themselves have set bad examples for some of the less mad who have been brought to the hospital." He cut them no slack, or anyone else. "At times, due to the fury and delusions of the masses in this State, it would have perhaps been difficult, if not impossible, for the most skillful psychologist to have determined who was sane or otherwise."

As you can see, W. P. did not suffer fools gladly.

By 1867 Tennessee had been restored to the Union for a year. Fisk University had opened and the Legislature had passed a law providing for separate schools for negroes at state expense. There were two hundred and seventy-one patients in the hospital: forty-seven had hereditary predispositions, twenty-six were there because of 'intemperance', and twenty-seven due to 'excitement incident to the war'. But things were getting better. The patients had 'decent coffee'. The buildings and farm were valued at three hundred thousand dollars.

A special building was erected on the grounds as a hospital for the colored insane: the Ewing Building. Having gained their freedom, deranged ex-slaves roamed the countryside. Dr. W. P. Jones acquired twenty-five thousand dollars from the legislature for the building, and later another seven thousand dollars for improvements. It may have been the first hospital to assure care for mentally ill African-Americans in the United States. W. P. praised the effort, "Tennesseans are the first people in the south to provide thus kindly and amply for a portion of their former servants."

A side note: Before the three-story brick building was razed in the '70s, I went through it with my dear friend Dr. Harold Jordan, the first African-American Commissioner of Mental Health in Tennessee.

In his 1867 report to the legislature, W. P. asked for money to build hospitals in Memphis and Knoxville as "those remote from a hospital are certainly neglected and a hospital in each division will remedy this evil." East Tennessee Hospital for the Insane opened in 1886 and West Tennessee Hospital for the Insane in 1889. This man is a lesson in what can be achieved if you have a plan and want it to happen, and what you can make happen if you refuse to give up.

With all these sweeping changes, W.P.'s eyes remained fixed on the here and now. One was to hire and retain good attendants. On one hand, if you hired a 'police force' type that would keep the place clean they tended to lack in gentleness. On the other, "those abounding in the milk of human kindness are usually too lazy or refined to attend to tables, beds, and water closets [commodes]."

> "Some of the patients sent to us are dangerous, [the attendants are not paid enough and] the best ones, after years with the insane are liable to become irritable or crabbed...many of our patients in the south, masters for example, men who have been in authority, accustomed to command, are more difficult to restrain under maniacal excitement. Last of all, perhaps few of us exhibit sufficient sympathy and respect for those who are devoting their lives to caring for the insane and can little know the cares, toils, tears, and risks that a faithful attendant goes through in caring for the insane."

Do you understand why I love him? Come hell or high water, Dr. W.P. spoke his beliefs and was always trying to make things better.

But he didn't soft sell the use of mechanical restraints. To keep an insane man from killing himself or someone else, he would use any and all methods of restraint at his disposal, such as sleeve jackets, leathern muffs, iron handcuffs, or the crib.

The last sentence in the report almost does not sound like him. But then, this multi-faceted man had a bit of religion in him and appreciated having survived a terrible time and was grateful that he himself was not insane, "Thankfully recognizing the providential protection which has kept us from 'the pestilence that walketh in darkness, and the destruction that wasteth at noon day', " I am,

W. P. Jones, M. D.
Superintendent

After the war, W. P. sent an itemized bill to "The Government of the United States" for nine thousand, one hundred and thirty yards of cedar fence; one hundred and five cords of wood; one hundred and thirty thousand bricks; sixty tons of clover hay; destruction of a flood gate; and some clothing for a guy named Lusky. He wanted four thousand, one hundred, and thirty dollars and received most of it.

Two years later W. P. resigned due to poor health after being hit on the head with a water pitcher by a patient. But his head was as hard as his tongue. He recovered and continued being a doctor and in time was elected to the state legislature—I bet he kept their feet to the fire—and then he helped found George Peabody College.

He was some kind of special! I'd like to have known him.

All the while W. P. was making things better, other advances were being made. Look back over what you have read and you will see the slow steady progress from David to Jesus to Green Grimes to Dorothea to W. P., and it has continued to this date.

Wars, all wars: the Revolutionary War, the Civil War, World War I, World War II, Korea, Vietnam, Iraq, Afghanistan kill and kill and kill: Little children, old people, husbands and wives are killed and gone forever. For those who survive nothing will be exactly the same again. So it was when our third son, Adam, was killed by a roadside bomb in Afghanistan in 2010. The hurt left behind for soldiers, families and civilians can be devastating: hopelessness, depression, rage, fear can turn inward to suicide or outward to murder of loved ones and others. From these wars came gradual recognition that mental illness is a national problem.

Here's what killing a Viet Cong soldier did to one Vietnam veteran, as told by Jonathan Shay in his book *Achilles in Vietnam*:

> "I just went crazy. I pulled him out into the paddy and carved him up with my knife. When I was done with him, he looked like a rag doll that a dog had been playing with...I lost my mercy. I felt a drastic

change after that...I couldn't do enough damage...For everyone I killed I felt better. Maybe some of the hurt went away. Every time you lost a friend, it seemed like a part of you was gone. Get one of them to compensate what they had done to me. I got very hard, cold, and lost all my mercy."[3]

The realization of the horrors of war has been present in every civilization. The Greeks included war within their words, 'Divine Madness'. A Civil War soldier said, "War is a living hell on earth." Yet knowing this doesn't stop us from killing over and over. These horrors have been present in every form: blood; fire; faces, arms and legs of friend and foe blown to bits; faiths suddenly needed and suddenly vanished; prayers that help one minute and fail the next. In the midst of roar and thunder, clash of sword and shell, horrors are born, some that overwhelm our very being. So it was with Yankees and Rebels between 1861 to 1865: six hundred twenty thousand died; three hundred sixty thousand from the North, two hundred sixty thousand from the South.

The American Civil War, as with all wars, not only injured many soldiers' bodies but also their minds. A description of Southern General James Longstreet after being wounded in the wilderness in May 1864 explains: "He says he does not see why a bullet going through a man's shoulder should make a baby of him." At home he was "very feeble and nervous...from his wound." And a Louisiana soldier, Will Pinkney, after defending New Orleans, became "woe begone, subdued, care-worn, and sad."

And there's the hero of Little Round Top at Gettysburg, General Governor Kemble Warren, who prevented disaster for the Union. With the mounting losses he became "irascible and unpredictable, his condition made worse by heavy drinking." On June 6, 1864, Colonel Wainwright described him, "He sleeps a great deal of the time, and says nothing to anyone. I think at times that these fits of his must be the results of a sort of insanity."

During World War I, an Australian soldier wrote home to his parents:

"You may be a little surprised to hear that I am in the hospital suffering from shell shock, which has taken my speech and hearing. It is some sixteen days now since it happened. We were in the trenches and going for dear life, when two of us spotted a German machine-gunner in a hole, so we made up our minds to have him, and I just remember getting to him when a high explosive shell burst at my head, it seemed as if it had burst inside my head, everything went black. I tried to call out and could not hear my mates—only just a terrible bursting in my head all the time. I never remembered anything more until I came onto the boat...the doctors think I will get alright in time."

Shell shock, the common diagnosis for major psychological reactions to battle in World War I, became battle fatigue in World War II. We now call it PTSD, Post Traumatic Stress Disorder. It can occur at any age and shows that anyone can develop a mental disorder given enough prolonged stress, such as the hell of war, or the abuse of a child; its potential lies within all of us. The following summary is taken from the 1994, *Diagnostic and Statistical Manual of Mental Disorders IV*, published by the American Psychiatric Association.

> "The essential feature of [PTSD] is the development of symptoms following exposure to an extreme traumatic exposure to an extreme traumatic stress ...[such as] military combat, violent personal assault (sexual, physical, robbery, mugging), being kidnapped, taken hostage, torture, natural disasters, sexually traumatic events, and many more. The trauma can be re-experienced...[in] recurrent and intrusive recollections...distressing dreams during which the event is replayed...events that resemble an aspect of the traumatic event, anniversaries of the event, etc."

One of my patients in Columbia was a combat veteran of Vietnam serving as a demolition expert who blew up underground tunnels. He came to see me in late fall, after seeing and smelling the flames and smoke from the burning off of sedge fields. The fire and smoke brought back the burning of villages, and the rattling sounds of logging trucks triggered memories of military trucks and armored carriers. It all came back again and again. In his bed at night he would see the flames and hear the screams of villagers. Maybe I helped him. I'm not sure. I hope so. Later on, I learned from his wife that he had become a member of the Ku Klux Klan.

Out of all the hell of war and its left-over remnants of damaged minds, there came an acknowledgment that we had to have more mental health services to help heal horrors that hadn't gone away. And—to our credit—we recognized that our understanding of mental illness was not only poor but, at times, incompetent. War, as with all disasters, personal or national, leave within their finalities things to learn—at times even for something better.

Early in the twentieth century the "mental hygiene" movement came into existence led largely by an intelligent, articulate man who had had hallucinations and paranoia resulting in hospitalization. When he came out of the hospital he was resentful and angry at what he had experienced and wrote a famous, graphic account of its degrading conditions. *The Mind that Found Itself* by Clifford Beers aroused those touched by mental illness and sparked a national movement to make improvements. It is still a book worth reading and from which much can be learned.

On the third day of July 1946, a progression into the future came with President Harry Truman signing the National Mental Health Act. It provided funding for psychiatric education and research and led to the creation in 1949 of the National Institute of Mental Health, a leader in supporting America's future treatment of neuropsychiatric disease.

In the early 1950s two giant strides forward were made with medications. The first was lithium, the second thorazine. Lithium was first used in the nineteenth century for the treatment of kidney and bladder disease and gallstones. Then, in 1870, it was used at Bellevue Hospital—the oldest public hospital in America—for acute mania. A Canadian Institutes of Health Research report stated, "The United States was more or less the last in-first out in using drugs other than lithium for bipolar patients. Finally, in the 1970s, convincing studies showed that lithium prevented relapses in depressive illness. The report also stated that, "With the exception of ECT (Electroconvulsive Therapy), lithium was the single most effective treatment in psychiatry." Now, many patients remain on lithium for decades.

Next came chlorpromazine. Most of us know it as thorazine. When it appeared in the early 1950s it was like a miracle drug for front-line psychiatrists treating patients who were severely psychotic. At the time, fifty percent of the people in psychiatric hospital beds throughout the world were suffering from schizophrenia with delusions, hallucinations, and jumbled behavior.

In 1952 Dr. Henri Laborit discovered thorazine, one of the first drugs to markedly reduce terrifying hallucinations, disturbing delusions, and agitation. It was so effective that beds and institutions for psychiatric patients declined sufficiently as community services expanded.

As helpful as these medications have been, they are not effective with everyone. For some patients the side effects are so unpleasant they refuse to take them.

Though not a scientist, I have long believed that research possesses the chisel and hammer for chipping away at the debilitations of severe mental illness, as is happening with cancer, heart, and other diseases. I believe the day will come when some of these illnesses will be preventable, as has occurred with polio and small pox.

A new generation of antipsychotic medications have been developed. Clozapine was the first. With minimal side effects when taking this drug, people with schizophrenia gradually began to regain their interest in life, their delusions and hallucinations decreased, and their thinking became clearer and more logical. It was developed by two American psychiatrists, Dr. John Kane and Dr. Herbert Meltzer. I came to know Dr. Meltzer in 1997 when we met at Vanderbilt Medical School to consider establishing a research relationship between Vanderbilt and the recently formed Centerstone, the largest mental health center in Tennessee. We began the research connection not long after. It continued until he left Vanderbilt and Tennessee. In 2016 he was presented with the Pioneer in Psychopharmacology Award at Northwestern University Feinberg School of Medicine.

Other antipsychotic medications have followed: Zyprexa, Seroquel and Zeldox. However, even these have their troubling side effects: increased appetite coupled with excessive weight gain and a tendency to develop diabetes.

And what about ECT? Though Electroconvulsive Therapy tends to scare people, I believe in its value. I assisted in giving shock treatment three times, twice at Central State Hospital in 1958, and once two years later at Vanderbilt. At Central State I helped patients onto the table, then held an arm and leg. On the other side of the table an aide held the other arm and leg. Electrodes were fixed on each temple and a small amount of electrical current was passed into the brain and the patient had a convulsion. I can still see the worried eyes when the tongue guard was put between their teeth to prevent them from biting their tongues and breaking teeth.

Much has improved in the administration of ECT. Now, anesthesia is given and the patient is usually asleep before the shock occurs.

With the exception of most clinicians, very few people have accurate information with a writing knowledge of ECT. So let me defend my positive judgment with some expert research. Read Nancy Coover Andreasen's *Brave New Brain: "Conquering Mental Illness in the Era of the Genome"* for her detailed explanation of how it is done and her summation that "ECT can be an extremely effective treatment for depression and sometimes for mania."

A statement by the National Institute of Mental Health further supports this method.

> "Electroconvulsive therapy is the best studied brain stimulation therapy and has the longest history of use...ECT is most often used to treat severe, treatment-resistant depression, but it may also be medically indicated in...bipolar disorder or schizophrenia. Two major advantages of ECT over medication are that ECT begins to work more quickly, often starting within the first week, and older individuals respond especially quickly.[4]

Another method of treatment is psychotherapy, what some call Talk Therapy. Its aim is to identify, understand and change emotions, thoughts, and behavior that are so troubling to the patient that they interfere with his life and sometimes the lives of others. I was a psychotherapist.

But so much more is involved than simply encouraging the troubled person to talk. There's listening, seeing and feeling–actively listening by the therapist—letting the patient know with your face and words that you hear him, you are attentive to him and are validating him and his feelings. When shared both ways, it is the heart and soul of trust, friendship, and love.

For many, if not all, there can be fear of asking for help, of crossing the doorstep, of walking into a room to talk with a stranger, a fear of telling hidden things that may be scowled upon or laughed at. There's a fear of telling things that, if known, might indicate the person is crazy or evil, or that in saying these things aloud might make them so. All the thoughts become so jumbled in the patient's head that he has no control over them or of his fear.

But the beginning of control and of healing can be the very formation of these jumbled thoughts and emotions into words and sentences, then saying them aloud to an understanding, trained person who does not scowl or judge.

Living a life, a full life, is filled with joy and laughter. For all of us there come hurts and tears and guilt. For some it can feel like damnation. Feelings of hopelessness, thoughts of suicide, fears and nightmares, loss of sleep and energy, no interest in love or love making, or work, or anything else—even eating. Then there comes a slow withdrawing from others, making the patient begin to slide backward into himself and into darkness.

Thank God, most of us are not alone and we're saved from ourselves by family and friends, some by belief in God and prayer, others by meditation and exercise, or by nature, art, music, and religion.

On an evening in the summer of 1958 a man was dying alone on the second floor of the men's ward in the Cooper Building at Central State Hospital where I worked. I called my wife and told her I would be late coming home because I was staying with a patient until he died. My reasons? I felt someone, even a stranger, should be with him. And I wanted to see what dying was like. He died a little after 10:00 p.m. that evening.

I hope I helped some of the people I saw find in themselves something that was already there to help them smile again. Maybe others found a bit of comfort for a while.

Yes, we've come a way and I am certain—at least, I believe—it will get better. But we are far from being there. Patients are still in jails and under bridges; the homeless are still wandering everywhere, maybe not as awful as in Dorothea Dix's day, but bad enough to remember her 1847 *Memorial for the Insane of the State of Tennessee*:

> "...Pining in cells and dungeons, pent in log cabins...now wandering at large, alone and neglected, endangering the security of property, often inimical to human life, and now thrust into cells...cast out, cast off...from comfort, hope, and happiness, such is the present

> actual condition of a large number of your fellow citizens, useless and helpless, life is at once grievous to themselves and a source of immeasurable sorrow to all beside [and especially to those who love them.]"[5]

Written one hundred sixty years ago to Tennessee, her words could have been written today.

In 1931, a building for the criminally insane was built and opened on the grounds of Central State Hospital. In that building an attorney taught me how to evaluate prisoners for competency in order to stand trial. It began with my going upstairs to a small room to interview a prisoner, followed by giving testimony to the attorney. I testified in court many times in my career, though not once for competency to stand trial—all were to give my recommendation for treatment.

VANDERBILT HOSPITAL
1960 to 1968

The Department of Psychiatry at the Vanderbilt School of Medicine was established in 1947. Thirteen years later the Children's Psychiatric Division opened. I was hired that same year to work as a psychiatric social worker and play therapist for the children's in-patient unit which treated children ages six through twelve. I could hardly believe it. Vanderbilt Hospital's Department of Psychiatry had actually hired me. I wore a white coat like a doctor. You could just about spit from my office to the office of the chairman of the department, Dr. William Orr. It was heady stuff.

I think it was in the movie, *Little Big Man*, that an old Indian says, "My heart soared like a hawk." Well, my heart soared like a hawk when I came to work in Child Psychiatry a few days before I graduated with my Master's degree from the University of Tennessee. The first Spain to graduate from college, then a Master's degree and I was going to work in Mecca (for me)—Vanderbilt. It made my parents proud and I made enough money for us to have a comfortable and lovely house. As you can tell, I still haven't recovered.

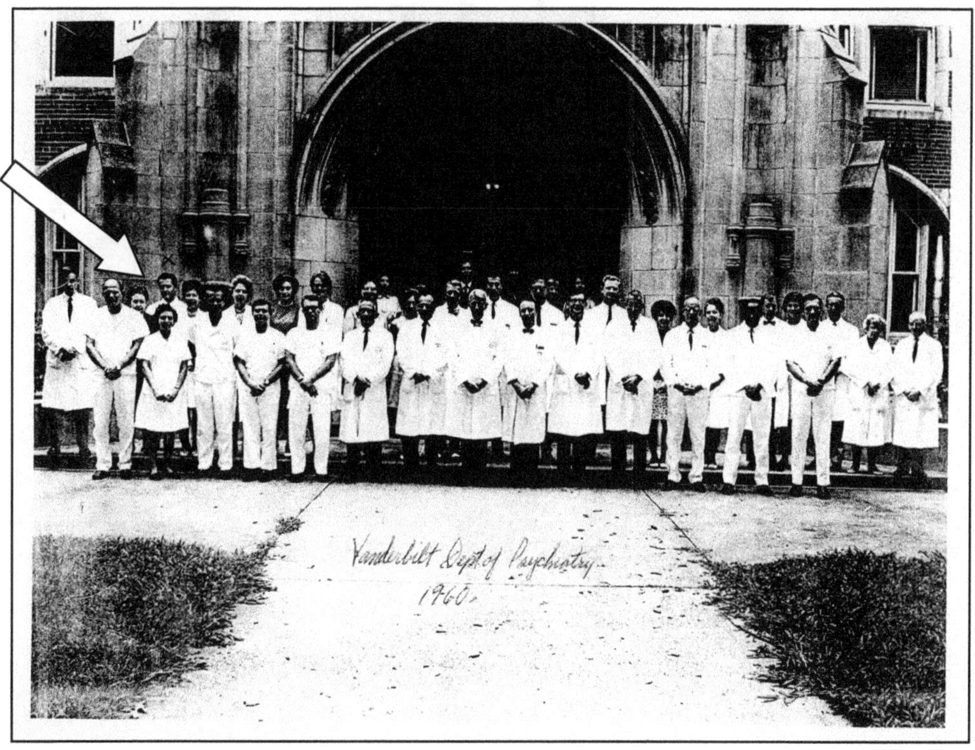

Vanderbilt Department of Psychiatry, 1960
George Spain is fourth from the left on the back row.

In the 1960s, in the Department of Psychiatry, you could smell Freud's cigar smoke, hear his listening silences as he scribbled notes sitting behind his reclining patient. Couches were everywhere. In fact, the office I was given had a nice one, which I soon traded to another psychiatrist for one of his comfortable, upright leather chairs. I believed then—and still believe—in Freud's method of taking us back into ourselves, into memories and dreams, into wherever our past leads.

the Staff . . .

1962

Most of the personnel of the Wills Center children's division are pictured above in a staff meeting. Acting Director Dr. H. James Crecraft is seated in the center. Others are, left to right, Dr. Charles Corbin, fellow in child psychiatry; Dr. James Gammill, child analyst; Clinton Griffin and William Boyd, teachers at the Wills Center School; Dr. John Pate, director of the School; George Spain, social worker; Mrs. Christine Fossick, teacher; Dr. Margaret Evans, child analyst; Miss Miriam McHaney, chief social worker; Miss Margaret Fernia, professor at the University of Tennessee School of Social Work, a visitor; Mrs. Bransford J. Norton, dietician; Miss Peggy Guess, nursing instructor; Mrs. Randolph Tucker, nursing supervisor; Janice Ricketson, social worker.

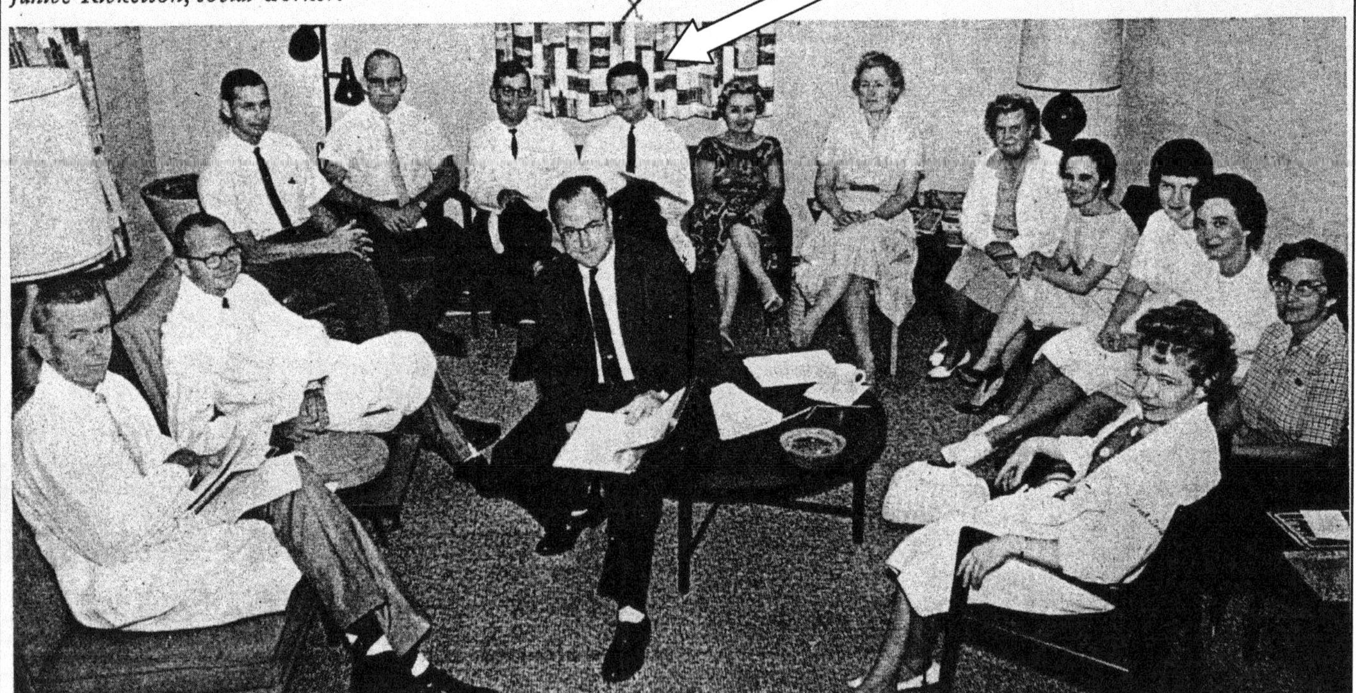

Psychoanalysis is a systematic attempt to understand the structure and actions of our inner world. Both a theory and a therapy, it shares borders with literature, medicine, psychiatry, and psychology.

First and foremost, its task is to soberly grapple with the demons of the irrational and then reduce these demons to words of understanding. Though many today proclaim Freud's message to be folderol, still we casually refer to his repression and projection, neurosis, ambivalence, and sibling rivalry.

On June 4, 1938 Freud and his family left Vienna to escape the Nazi purge of Jews. Helped by several analysts, they arrived in London a few days later. A year later Britain and France declared war on Germany. Still smoking his cigars Freud died of cancer of the mouth at three in the morning on September 23, 1939.[6]

Before moving on let me say I strongly believe in some of Freud's theories and practices. History lives on inside the genes and memories of each of us. Rippling down from our great, great grandparents, great grandparents, grandparents, and parents, our pasts leave their marks on all of us. Faulkner said it in clearer words than Freud,

> "Tomorrow is just another name for today."
> "...But tomorrow is today also."
> "Yao. Tomorrow is today."
>
> "History is not was. It is."

But I also believe—I know—we are more, much more, than our pasts in memories and our unconscious. We are all born with "warts" inside and outside, some big, some small. Not one of us came out perfect; otherwise, we'd all live forever, and though not one of us has as yet pulled this off, many believe we do. We are all made up of bits and pieces of what we call genes and DNA that twist and turn in us in ways that can be strange and wonderful and painful to us as well as to others. In part, it is what this book is about.

Once in harness at Vanderbilt, surrounded by thoroughbreds, I pulled like a plow mule. Patiently, they helped me rise above my ignorance. Gradually, I began to know what I was doing. Eventually, I became good at it. I had some of the best clinical supervisors in the United States. Each one was a good person.

Margaret Gwen Evans, PhD, an entomologist, as well as a psychoanalyst, specialized in treating young children and was one of my clinical supervisors. Like my mother's father she was Welsh. As an entomologist she had worked in India. Nehru had been one of her students in London; and in India, she had heard one of my heroes, Gandhi, speak. Illness brought her home. Never married, her neat, polite, intelligent, attentive manner might have caused you to think she was an old maid schoolteacher. She had met Freud in the Freuds' London home a number of times while training with Anna, Sigmund's analyst daughter, who was an imminent child analyst.

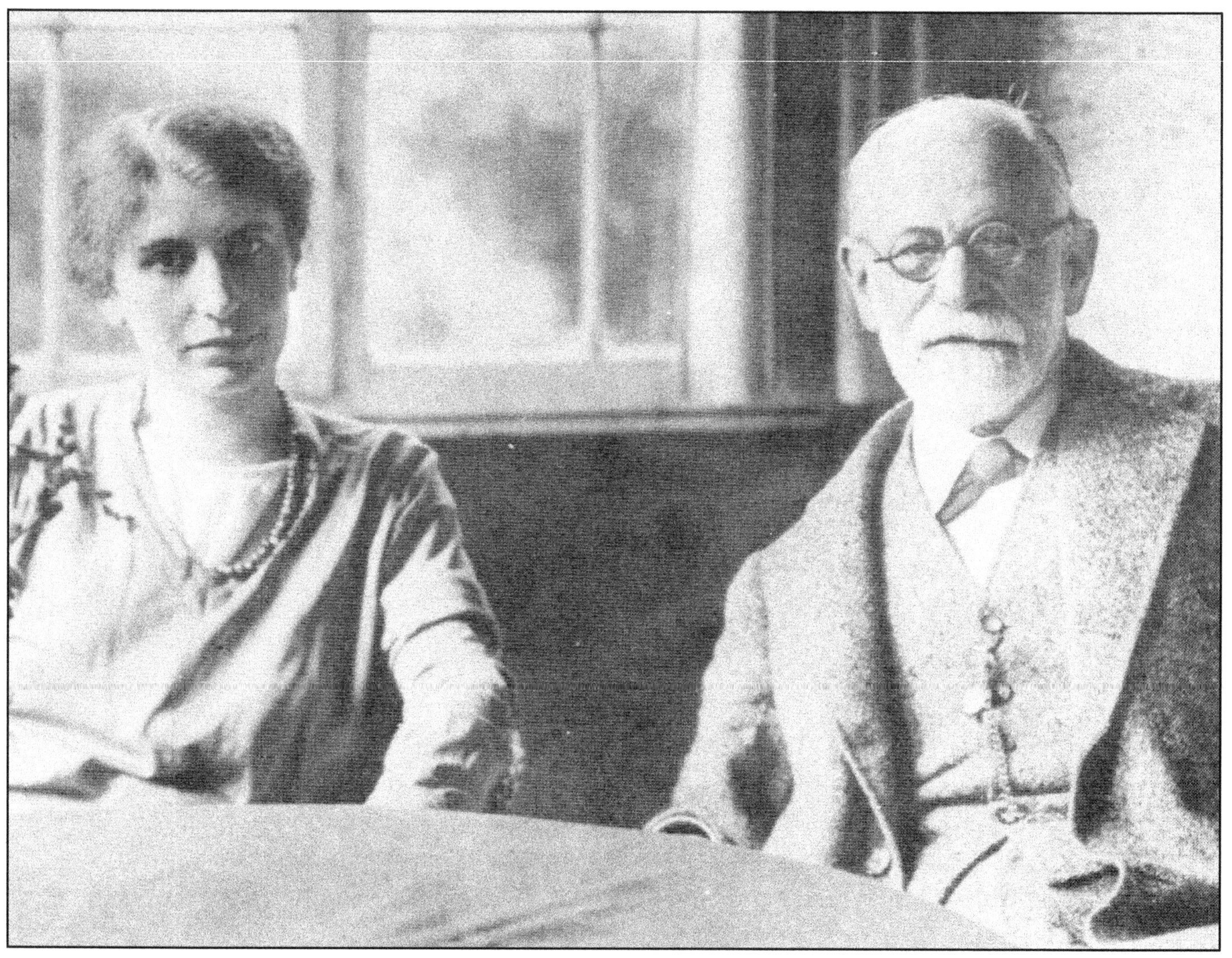

Freud with Anna in the fall of 1928.

In contrast to my meandering mind and ways, Dr. Evans always seemed precise and in full control with what I imagined was a touch of Victorianism. Yet, she had roamed India, Australia and the United States on her own. In Australia, during her younger years she had been a governess on a sprawling sheep ranch, where she first learned of Freud and decided to become an analyst.

When I knew Dr. Evans she was a member of the British Psychoanalytical Society.

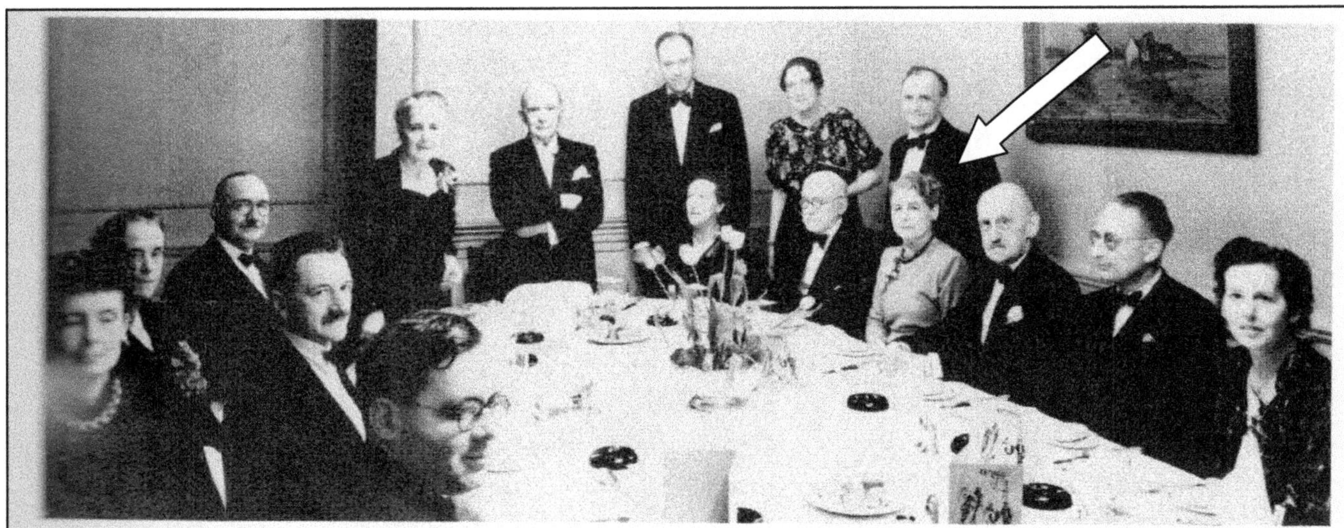

Dinner to celebrate Melanie's 70th birthday in 1952. From left: (seated) Marion Milner, Sylvia Payne, W. Clifford M. Scott, Roger Money-Kyrle, Eric Clyne; (standing) Melanie Klein, Ernest Jones, Herbert Rosenfeld, Joan Riviere, Donald Winnicott; (seated) Paula Heimann, James Strachey, Gwen Evans, Cyril Wilson, Michael Balint, Judy Clyne.

Having no family of her own in Nashville, she practically adopted my family as her own. She often asked Jackie and me to assist in her small supper gatherings of seven. Jackie helped in the kitchen and I served the booze: libations of scotch whiskey and sherry for the talk before the food and then merlot. The small gatherings were mostly composed of psychiatrists, analysts, and an anthropologist.

I had another unmarried supervisor, James "Jim" Gammill, M.D., child analyst. Born in Flat Creek, Tennessee he'd served as a navigator in World War II and participated in the liberation of France. Kind, soft-voiced, drenched in manners and ways of the Old South, he bought a farm with a two-story white-frame antebellum house that he named "Cleburne Hall". We adopted him and he adopted us—all seven of us.

Like Dr. Evans, he was cultured, neat, and polite. Were all analysts like that? If I remember correctly, he was a Presbyterian, or he could have been Methodist. Whichever, if he had dressed in a black suit instead of a white lab coat you might have thought he was one of those friendly, very smart ministers you would like to know.

After completing his medical studies in the United States, he returned to Europe and trained from 1950 to 1960 as a psychoanalyst, part of this training with Melanie Klein and Dr. W. Winnicott, two of the world's leading therapists for emotionally disturbed children.

In 1966 he returned to Europe to live in Paris where he became a leader in developing skills of the full range of psychoanalysis—children, adolescents, and adults. He invited Jackie and me to come stay with him at his home outside Paris but, alas, we never did. Our friend and one of my best teachers died in 2017 at the age of ninety-two.

Miss Miriam McHaney was my wonderful social work supervisor, a short, stocky, unmarried woman with a ruddy, smiling face. I never knew if she was Scots or Irish. I chose Irish because of her look and way. I loved her being a fine violinist who played with the Nashville Symphony. She had been Mary Hemingway's good friend and hung out with her and Ernest in Parisian cafes. She once told me that whenever you were with him and the two of you were talking, no matter the hubbub going on around you, he was totally focused on you, listening and watching your eyes and face. Hemingway describes his love for Paris in his *A Moveable Feast*.

> "In the early days writing in Paris I would invent not only from my own experience but from the experiences and knowledge of my friends and all the people I had known, or met since I could remember, who were not writers. I was very lucky that all my best friends were not writers and to have known many intelligent people who were articulate."

So the unanswered question still comes to me: Is Miss McHaney part or parcel of one of his stories?

Though offered the opportunity to train at the Tavistock Institute in London for three years to become a lay analyst, I turned it down after deciding with Jackie that it might lead to our never returning to Nashville where our lives were interwoven with family and friends. What we might gain was so much less than what we might lose.

COLUMBIA, TENNESSEE
1968 to 1992

Rather than London, I went to Columbia, Tennessee in 1968 to work at the fledgling Maury County Mental Health Clinic. Thank God, for these were to be the best years of my career. We lived in Williamson County, just thirty miles away.

At the beginning, there were five of us: Dr. Dave Shupe, Psychiatrist-Director, who I had known at Vanderbilt during his residency; a psychological examiner who, thus far, had only performed social security evaluations; two office staff; and myself. We occupied the second floor of the old post office. Entering a side door you went up narrow steps to a fair-sized waiting room with narrow halls leading to several offices. All the walls were a faded army-green. The first time I saw it I said it looked like a place where illegal abortions might have once been performed. But the board members were everything you would hope for to help start mental health services in a rural area. They were the leaders of the county, most especially County Judge John Stanton, a lawyer and former F.B.I. agent.

Everything in my personal and professional life came together in Maury County, the surrounding counties, and the farms and forests stretching south and east and west. My own people were country people who'd fed their families and made their livings off tobacco, hogs, and corn (Did I mention corn whiskey?), and hard work. I loved every minute of it—well, almost—the thirty years I was there. There were times when it was like a barroom brawl. We were good at what we did. We saw people at night, in jails, and in schools over eight counties. At first, we saw a hundred people, then two hundred, then a thousand, then more and more. And we hired more and more staff to help us.

After two years Dr. Shupe left for Oklahoma. Dr. Orr was retiring from the Chairmanship of the Department of Psychiatry at Vanderbilt and, when I went to his office to ask him if he knew a psychiatrist that might replace Dr. Shupe, he said, "How about someone with one foot in the grave?" And I'll be damned! He meant himself! I was blessed to have him come and become our director who led us on our next giant stride forward.

He was a clinician's clinician, attentive to minute details of his patients. He listened carefully to their tellings and, in turn, used their words and ways to let them know he understood and, at the same time, he was unerring regarding their medication needs. You could tell by his very being that he was a patrician. Anyone would enjoy going into St. Peter's Episcopal Church, built in 1860, on West Seventh in Columbia to see the two fine stained glass Orr Windows installed by his ancestors. The church stands across the street from the Memorial Building where the Maury County Clinic is located.

He was always teaching. One day he came to the open door of my office with an elderly black man behind him. "George, have you got a minute?"

"Yes, sir, come in."

He stepped in followed by the man, a patient he had just seen, "George, this is Mr. Turner. Mr. Turner, this is Mr. Spain. Mr. Turner has been depressed and is kind enough to let me show you his rare skin disorder. Mr. Turner, would you mind pulling up your sleeve and showing Mr. Spain your arm?" The man pulled up his sleeve and I was looking at what looked like alligator hide. I don't think I jerked back or let my face look repelled. "Mr. Turner, can Mr. Spain reach over and feel your arm?"

"Yes, sir," he said.

As I moved my hand over it, Dr. Orr was telling me the cause and course of the disease though I heard none of it as I felt and stared at the rough skin. Then Dr. Orr asked, "George, I wonder if you could help Mr. Turner find some teeth so he could eat corn on the cob again, which he thinks will help him feel better."

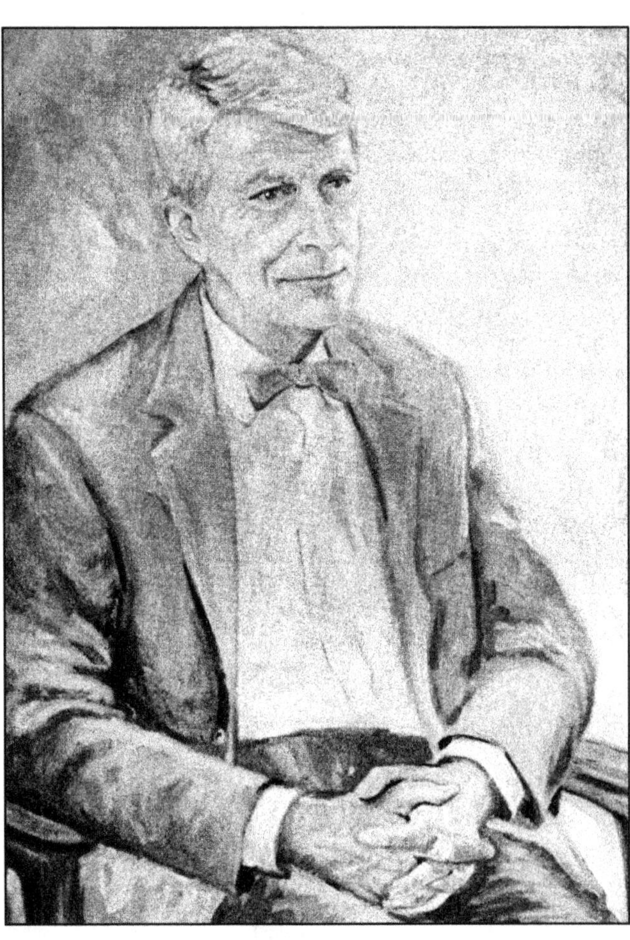

"Yes, sir," I said. Eventually, with the help of Meharry Hospital's Dental School, Mr. Turner got his teeth.

And so it was that a day might pass in a rural mental health clinic.

When Dr. Orr became our director, the first thing he did was to go to Central State Hospital once a week for an entire day to evaluate every patient from our eight counties. There were dozens upon dozens and he saw them all.

From these evaluations we prepared the way for many to be released and come home or, at least, moved to facilities nearer to their homes, where we could care for them. As I write this and remember it, tears fill my eyes. I can see an orange-ish school bus coming toward our center filled with people from the State hospital where they had lived many long years. A few families were waiting to accept their loved ones. Nursing homes took the others. We oversaw their psychiatric medications for long years afterwards. I cannot recall any of the patients returning to the State hospital.

Dr. Orr retired as Executive Director of the Columbia Area Mental Health Center in 1974. The board accepted his recommendation and asked me to be the new director. I held the position until February 1997 when I became the CEO of Pinnacle Health Center.

Before moving on, I want to say some last words about Dr. Orr. After a stroke in 1983 he went steadily downhill. Mrs. Orr was exhausted from caring for him at home and their children lived out of state. I called her one day and asked if she would like to take a rest and visit their summer home in Maine. We could arrange to care for him at Graymere Nursing Home in Columbia. We arranged this, oversaw all his medical needs and visited him daily. He died there on Monday, November 28, 1983. I kissed him and said, "I love you," two hours before he died. Maury County's newspaper, The Daily Herald, printed my tribute the next Friday. Here is a small bit of it:

> "He had qualities similar to Samuel Johnson, one of which Boswell gives in his Life of Samuel Johnson, 'His superiority over other learned men consisted chiefly in what may be called the art of thinking, the art of using the mind, a certain continual power of seizing the useful substance of all that he knew and exhibiting it in a clear and forceful manner.'"
>
> "He once told me, 'I would much rather smell the odor of good honest sweat, than expensive perfume.'" And 'you must always focus on the needs of the individual.'"

Twice we crossed swords. He won the first bout. I won the second.

CENTERSTONE
1997 to 2000

Early in 1997 Pinnacle Health was formed by Columbia Area, Harriett Cohn (Clarkesville area) and Highland Rim (Tullahoma area) mental health centers, covering twenty counties in middle Tennessee. Later the same year, Centerstone was created through a merger between Pinnacle Health and the large, long-established Dede Wallace Center in Nashville. Things were happening quickly. As CEO, my clinical time was gradually eaten away by administrative meetings, speeches, working on legislation, and driving and driving. I saw fewer and fewer people that we were there to help. But those I did see helped keep me abreast of and anchored by what we were supposed to be about. Hours, days, and nights at work began to overwhelm my hours at home with my family.

Yet, I look back with mostly joy as we built Centerstone. Now located in several states, it serves over one hundred thousand people a year, has become the largest mental health center in the United States, and makes a major commitment to research.

Every day in 1954, Tennessee had seven thousand three hundred patients in four state hospitals.[7] The hospitals had become warehouses just piling up patients. Once admitted, some did not get better and lived the remainder of their lives there, dying there, and many being buried there.

Between the 1960s and 1997 mental health services spread like kudzu across Tennessee as they did across the nation. Following are chronological successes and failures of those years, sprinkled with some personal observations.

Message from the President of the United States
relative to
MENTAL ILLNESS AND MENTAL RETARDATION

"It is my intention to send shortly to the Congress a message pertaining to this Nation's most urgent needs in the area of health improvement...mental illness and mental retardation.

"Nearly one-fifth of the two hundred and seventy-nine State mental institutions are fire and health hazards; three-fourths of them were opened before World War I.

> "Nearly half of the five hundred and thirty thousand patients in our State mental hospitals are in institutions with over three thousand patients, where individual care and consideration are almost impossible.
>
> "Many of these institutions have less than half the professional staff required—with less than one psychiatrist for every three hundred and sixty patients.
>
> "Forty-five percent of their inmates have been hospitalized for ten years or more.
>
> "Central to a new mental health program is comprehensive community care...These centers will...provide better community care...to serve the mental health needs of the community.
>
> "We as a nation have long neglected the mentally ill and the mentally retarded."
>
> John F. Kennedy
> The White House
> February 5, 1963

The old Davidson County Psychiatric Hospital was closed in 1964. Some of its six hundred patients were transferred to nursing homes, but most of them were transported to Central State Hospital. Fifteen community mental health centers had been established in the state.

Twenty years later, the daily number in the state hospitals had dropped to one thousand, seven hundred and fifty-three. There were thirty-three centers with eighty-five clinics in Tennessee's ninety-five counties. Patients from our eight counties had plummeted from four hundred and twenty a day to thirty-three.[7]

Deinstitutionalization was doing what it was supposed to as it shifted patients away from hospitals to community care. Things were better in many ways but there were still problems, big ones, major ones. More and more, newspaper articles and letters to the editor criticized the increasing numbers of mentally ill people on the streets, sleeping and eliminating under bridges and in parks, begging and behaving in strange, sometimes frightening ways. More and more they were showing up in jails. It seemed almost that the ghost of Dorothea Dix's day was returning.

For too many, too much was missing: shelter, food, clothing, hygiene, medication, guidance, and some form of affection or at least some recognition as fellow humans. Some had been rejected by their families. Though they had a freedom of sorts, the debilitating effects of their illnesses kept them from little more than a day-to-day existence. Those of us who provided community mental health services were failing them. We needed to do more: more looking at ourselves, our priorities, our listening to and learning from those with the illnesses and their families. Along with state departments of mental health and community mental health centers, we all needed to accept part of the blame for those living under bridges, wandering the streets, and those who were locked up.— "They are us."

Mental health associations, the Alliance for the Mentally Ill—founded by families in 1979—and investigative news reporters put the spurs to us to fund a range of community support services needed by "those on the streets."

A Staff Writer for the *Tennessean* wrote on September 25, 1988:

> "For the past six years ["Two Step"] has lived in an alley behind the [Nashville Union Rescue] mission, taking his meals from a nearby dumpster and sleeping inside the mission only if the weather turns bitterly cold.
>
> "An advocate for the homeless familiar with Two Step says the man needs treatment for severe mental illness, but he cannot be hospitalized—according to state law—unless he seeks treatment on his own or the court commits him because he is violent to himself or others.
>
> "Advocates for improved mental health services argue that cases like the one above are stark evidence that the state's delivery system of care for the seriously mentally ill is inadequate.
>
> "Nationwide the National Alliance for the Mentally Ill estimated that there were two million persons who were seriously mentally ill, the vast majority suffering from schizophrenia or manic-depressive illness."

Ten years later, on March 7, 1999, *Tennessean* reporter Ellen Dahnke wrote, "Jail as Mental Ward." It exemplifies good journalism. It was critical and correct. Following are excerpts and summations:

> They perch and scream on the sidewalk, maybe even accost people from time to time. They are unkempt and unloved by business owners while passersby mutter they ought to be in jail.
>
> In Tennessee, they likely will eventually be locked up. They are not criminals. Many are mentally ill. About the only place to put them is jail.
>
> The law states that no person can be institutionalized unless he or she presents "an immediate danger to himself or others."
>
> "We've got to do something better than we're doing," said [George] Spain. "And for the first time law enforcement, mental health professionals, families and state officials are talking together."
>
> "Jails are not mental hospitals, and they shouldn't be in the business. We have a chance to find something better," said Jeff Blum, a mental health advocate.

The article offered a glimmer of hope along with a statewide survey of jails conducted in 1998 by the Tennessee Mental Health Planning Council and the Governor's Title 33 Commission. Governor Don Sundquist appointed the twenty-seven member Commission to comprehensively review and revise the mental health code for the improvement of Tennessee mental health and mental retardation services. I was one of them.

The Planning Council's survey of eighty-three jails out of the ninety-eight in Tennessee found almost one of every five inmates were believed to have some form of mental illness—totaling almost four thousand.

The Commission met monthly through 1999 reviewing Tennessee's existing mental health laws. We submitted our findings and recommendations to the Governor in January 2000. A few months later, "the General Assembly passed the most sweeping changes to laws governing the mentally ill in this state in thirty-five years." [*Tennessean*, Editor's Page, July 1, 2000]

Summary of Major Changes Brought About by the Law

- Name of the department was changed to the Department of Mental Health and Developmental Disabilities.
- Significantly expanded regulatory authority.
- Extended criminal background checks to mental health provider employees.
- Extended eligibility for people with developmental disabilities.
- Extended licensure requirements for supported living facilities.
- Required regular regimented planning and updating.
- Established a statewide council with a majority of members being consumers.
- Provided for services that would be provided by designated entities.
- Provided for surrogates to make decisions for adults with developmental disabilities due to mental impairment.
- Permitted in-patient services for up to seventy-two hours without judicial proceedings for persons with severe impairments when the need for psychiatric service was certified by two psychiatrists.
- Permitted mandatory community service for up to two years for persons charged with felonies, who were incompetent to stand trial, and not committable.
- Created special provision for children and their families.
- Allowed for advanced directives by consumers for their care.

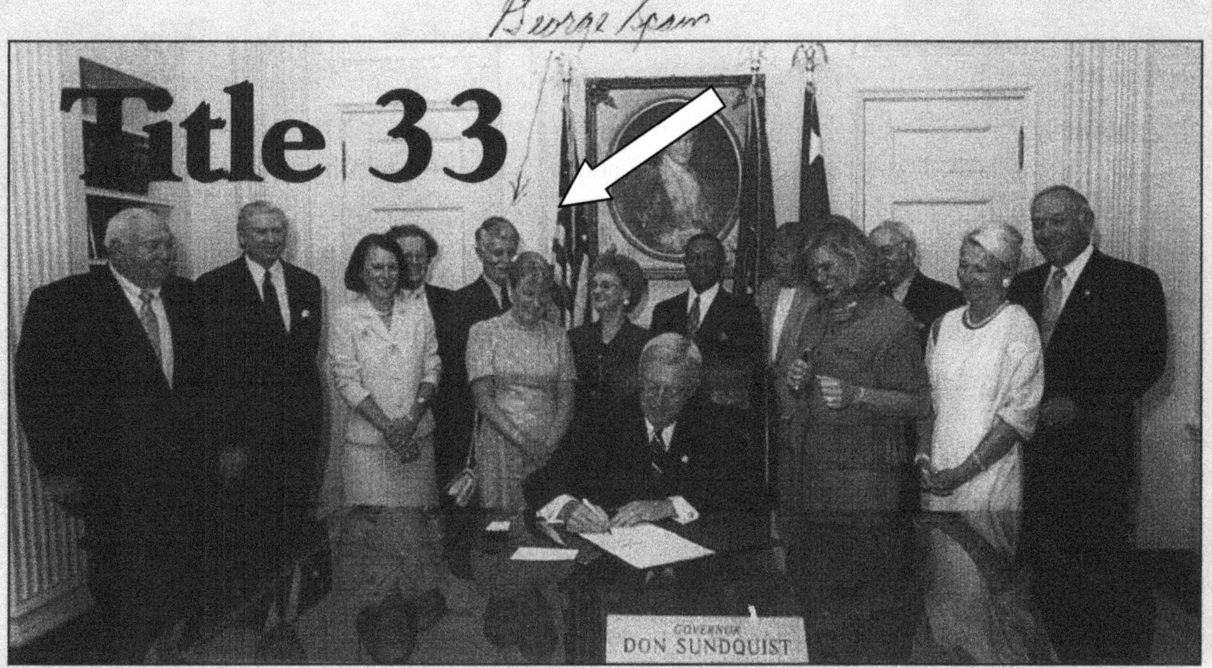

Happy Day: Advocates and state officials watch as Governor Don Sundquist signs into law revisions to Title 33 of the Tennessee Code Annotated. Pictured from left to right: Andy Fox, C. Richard Treadway, M.D., Mary Rolando, Grayford Gray, George Spain, Elisabeth Rukeyser, June Palmer, Governor Don Sundquist, Evelyn Robertson, Carol Westlake, Rep. Mary Ann Eckles, Gaylon Booker, Debi Tate and Ben Dishman.

On June 23, 2000, Governor Don Sundquist signed into law a total revision of Title 33 of the Tennessee Code Annotated—the area that governs the delivery of services to Tennesseans with mental illness, serious emotional disturbance, developmental disabilities and persons who need in-patient alcohol and/or drug services.

Prior to 1953, when Tennessee began providing residential and treatment services under the Department of Mental Health (as it was then called), mental health care was the responsibility of the State Board of Control, State Board of Administration and Institutions.

Original laws governing the provision of services primarily focused on making things expedient for government and care providers - not on the personal needs of individuals. In those days, Tennessee did not necessarily adopt a "people first" approach.

The revision, which unanimously passed both houses of the legislature, set the tone for service delivery for the future that reflected in the name change to the Department of Mental Health and Developmental Disabilities (DMHDD).

Under the law's provisions, the DMHDD must plan for and promote the availability of a comprehensive array of high quality prevention, early intervention, treatment and rehabilitation services and supports based on the needs and choices of service recipients and families served.

The new law expands, significantly, the DMHDD's regulatory authority and the people who are eligible for services; requires all providers to meet basic quality standards and all licensees to have conflict resolution procedures; makes the department more accountable; includes families and consumers in all aspects of the planning, developing and monitoring of service systems; and extends the rights of service recipients to the total service system.

Following are other significant changes to the law:

- Requires ongoing programs and budget planning effort; involves service recipients; makes programs subject to appropriations.
- Mandates cooperation with other agencies.
- Fills service gaps—mandatory services, three-day admissions.
- Gives service recipient role in care through advance directives.
- Creates Chapter Eight with special provisions for children and families—sets guiding principles, requires interagency agreements and interdepartmental planning for services by more than one agency.
- Provides monitoring of services without walls.

In 2003, the DMHDD will celebrate its 50th year. The passage of time has brought many changes in treatment concepts. One concept dictates that the kind of care provided be in the hands of providers and based on available resources. The other - the one supported by the new legislation - looks at the total person and family, encourages a comprehensive approach to services and gives the service recipient and his family a say into all aspects of the service system.

For further information on Title 33, go to the following internet address: www.state.tn.us/mental/t33/PC947unofficialcompilation.pdf

Breakthrough, Tn Dept MH/MR, June 2002

Much good has come from these changes. And yet as I sit here writing in June 2018, in front of me is that longtime mental health advocate, Tipper Gore's full page November 2017, article in the *Tennessean*: "*America's mental health system is fragile and needs careful treatment*." She states that, "Mental illness and substance abuse have reached crisis proportions. Too many Americans—especially young adults—live undiagnosed and untreated. One in five experience a mental illness, yet only twenty percent get help. Suicide is now the second leading cause of death among fifteen- to twenty-four-year-olds—recently surpassing car accidents."

In October 2017, the *Tennessean* reported that the Mental Health Cooperative had plans to establish a "psychiatric emergency room" in Nashville. For years the Cooperative had provided services to Nashville's Metro Jail and, along with Centerstone, had been the largest mental health provider in middle Tennessee.

The goals of the new service are to increase services to those in crisis, and to "make it easier for police to drop off someone mentally ill without criminal charges...and enable the officer to get back on the street in ten minutes".

Pam Womack, a longtime mental health colleague of mine has been the CEO of the Cooperative since it's founding in 1993. She tells me the new emergency service will open in early 2019. Hopefully, this along with other improved medications and services from Centerstone and other providers will make a dent in some of our past failures.

From their beginnings, mental health centers have responded to emergencies and disasters in their communities. Here's a few we dealt with in the eight counties served by the Columbia Area Mental Health Center.

- In March 1973, the Duck River flooded. One-fifth of Columbia was under water. Large parts of Maury County were totally surrounded by water. Three hundred families were evacuated. The governor called up the National Guard for search and rescue. The clinic was on high ground three blocks from the river and was not in danger. Four of us went to help the Guard. We were assigned to military trucks and spent the day evacuating families.
- On the weekend of June 28, 1977 a fire at the Maury County jail killed thirty-six inmates and six visitors. Mike Jean, one of our staff who worked with alcohol- and drug-addicted inmates, rushed to the jail and offered our center as a morgue if needed. Thankfully, it was not needed,

but he brought in the horrified families and provided counseling and support.

- In December 1986 a Lawrence County boarding home serving mentally ill people burned to the ground. Seven died. Our staff provided support and follow-up treatment.
- In February 1987 a second boarding home for the mentally ill and homeless in Lawrence County burned to the ground. We helped arrange for twenty-seven of the residents to be housed in a motel. The Center was recognized by Governor McWherter and the House of Representatives for its immediate response to the fire.
- On August 24, 1992, Hurricane Andrew devastated southern Florida, leaving fifty-two dead, two hundred fifty thousand homeless, sixty-three thousand destroyed homes, no power for one and a quarter million homes, and twenty billion dollars in damages. Several of my fellow directors and I put together four professional teams, including one psychiatrist. Each team went, one at a time, for a week into Homestead, the center of relief operations. For most of our time there, my wife and I worked in the tent city with young children. Four Tennessee centers contributed to these teams: Harriett Cohn, Vanderbilt, Luton, and Columbia.
- In May 1995 a Lawrence County tornado killed three people. The Center provided counseling.
- On November 15, 1995 a shooting occurred at Richland High School in Lynnville, Giles County Tennessee. A student with a .22-calibre rifle killed another student and a teacher. Within two hours we had a counselor at the school to help, and soon after made arrangements with a Church of Christ in Pulaski for our counselors to meet there with students and families.

Once a month for three years, one of our staff drove from Columbia through miles and miles of forest in Hickman County to evaluate prisoners at Turney Center for Youthful Offenders. We helped during a period of racial conflict in the Maury County school system. We consulted with the courts and legislators. We assisted in the creation of new social and health agencies and helped in the development of state mental health laws and policies. We raised funds for needed services, built clinical buildings and created affiliations between centers. Speeches galore were given to educate the community, state leaders, and politicians.

As I look back on those years I remember how the good far outweighed the bad. And how much they taught me about the joyful and the painful existence of living. I'm filled with memories of faces, names, places, struggles, anxieties, and laughter. And I hear Churchill's almost biblical words during the midst of World War II, "Never give in, never, never, never, never–in nothing, great or small, large or petty–never give in except to convictions of honor and good sense...continue to pester, nag, and bite."

For all of us, life is filled with whacks. Some come before we're born, some later, some keep on coming. Some make us cry or fill us with rage until we want to give up. Some of us pray, some of us curse. Some hurt others, some shoot themselves or take overdoses. Some say, "To hell with it," spit on the ground, and walk away.

I hear these words from my Aunt Virginia, "George Edward, when I start gettin' what I guess people call 'down', I put on a dixieland jazz record an' dance 'round the house. An' if that doesn't help, I go into the bathroom an' look in the mirror an' laugh my butt off."

That's real wisdom! So from me to you, go laugh your butt off!

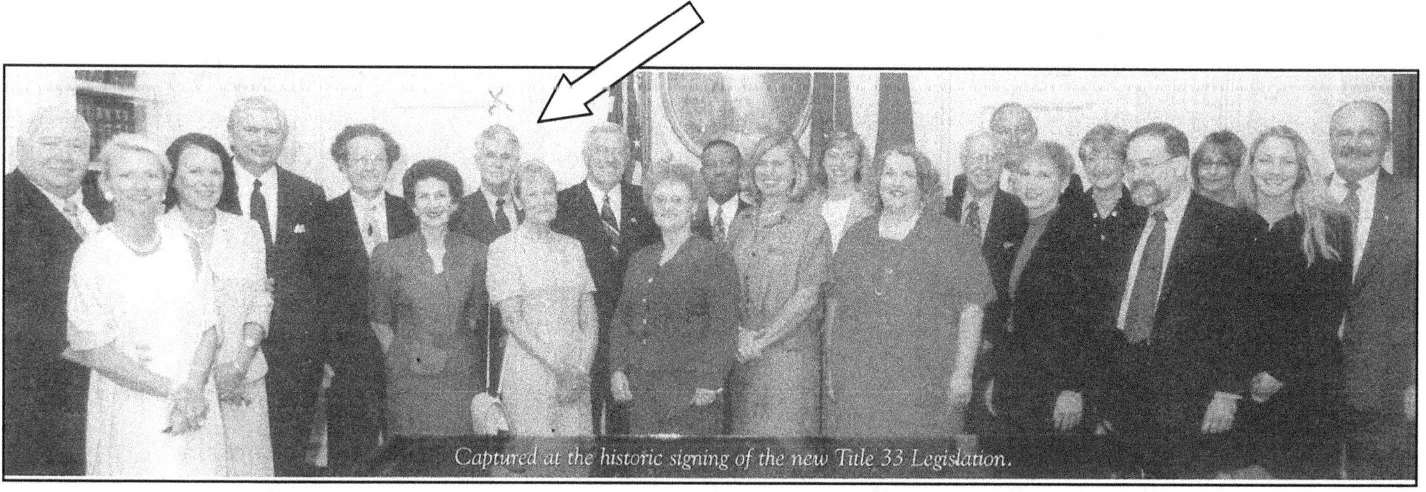

Captured at the historic signing of the new Title 33 Legislation.

EPILOGUE

I retired in 2003 and took up writing with a vengeance. While I loved my work, my life, thank God, has been filled with more—much more: Jackie, our five children, thirteen grandchildren, five great grandchildren, wonderful in-laws, and a host of friends who have given me their love, joy, and support through good times and bad.

Jackie died in 2009. A year later, our third son, Adam, was killed in Afghanistan. The pain from their deaths remains within me; every week I cry a moment or two for them. I live in the same house where Jackie died and where Adam's belongings were returned.

Authoring twelve books, a bunch of short stories, performing readings all over middle Tennessee and associating with some fine writers who have become my friends have helped lift me up. Several of the stories and characters I have created have risen from my personal joys and grief.

> *"Think of all that has happened here, on this earth. All the hot and strong for living, pleasuring, that has soaked back into it. For grieving and suffering too, of course, but still getting something out of it, getting a lot out of it. After all, you don't have to continue to bear what you believe is suffering; you can always choose to stop and put an end to it. And even suffering and grieving is better than nothing. There is only one thing that's worse than not being alive, and that's shame. But you can't be alive forever, and you always wear out life long before you have exhausted the possibilities of living. And all that must be somewhere; all that could not have been invented and created just to be thrown away..."*
>
> William Faulkner
> *The Big Woods*

NOTES

1. Charles Bailey Bell, *The Bell Witch of Tennessee*, 1934, Charles Elder, Publisher, Nashville, Tennessee.
2. Paul Dokecki and Janice Mashburn, *Beyond the Asylum: The History of Mental Handicap Policy in Tennessee*, 1984, Tennessee Department of Mental Health and Mental Retardation.
3. Michael Adams, *Living Hell: The Dark Side of the Civil War*, 2014. Most of the information on pages 37 and 38 is taken from *Living Hell.*
4. Nancy Coovers Andreasen, M.D., Ph.D., *Brave New Brain: Conquering Mental Illness in the Era of the Genome*, Oxford University Press, Publisher, 2001.
5. Dorothea Dix, *Memorial for the Insane of the State of Tennessee*, 1847, Tennessee State Archives.
6. Elizabeth Roundinesco, *Freud in His Time and Ours*, 2016, Harvard University Press.
7. Tennessee Department of Mental Health and Mental Retardation reports.

PART TWO

STORIES OF MENTAL ILLNESS

DEATH OF A CONFEDERATE CAPTAIN

This story originated with a photograph of my wife's great grandfather, William Lynch and his two brothers, Francis and Lafayette, who fought with him in the First Tennessee Infantry during the Civil War. Francis was killed at William's side at the Battle of Kennesaw Mountain. William wrote to their parents in Winchester, Tennessee telling where he had buried Francis. A few years ago I gave this letter in William's handwriting to the Tennessee State Archives. The following story has been changed to the death of a son beside his father and the guilt of the father for being unable to save his son.

They said Captain Robert Taggert hanged himself in Lady's stall, on June 27, 1874, because she had been his son, Bob's, favorite saddle horse. Bob had died on that exact same day, ten years before. Years later, Aunt Sally, the Taggert's cook, told me that the rope broke after the Captain was dead and that his body fell into the straw but the mare never stepped on him. Though he didn't leave a note, I knew why the "Captain," for that's what everybody called him, did what he did.

My mother had tried to heal the Captain, but it didn't help. In fact, something she did may have played a part in his death. That's what Mrs. Taggert and her sons and her brother, John Gaunt, the high sheriff of Franklin County, believed. After the Captain died, they said Mama was a witch. His death made a sadness in me because he was a good man and for a while I had imagined him as my father. But before it was all over, the greatest sadness of my life came to me.

Mama was a red-headed Irish immigrant born with the veil over her face and the gift of healing. Her eyes were gray and shaped like a deer's. I thought she was beautiful. Practically everything that is good in me came from her, for I never knew my father, Joseph. I was a baby when he was killed charging with the colored troops up Peach Orchard Hill at the Battle of Nashville. She told me that he was born a slave in Georgia and that he killed his master with a sickle. Then he fled north into the mountains near Sewanee.

In a valley, called Lost Cove, he was bitten by a rattlesnake. My mother, who lived in the valley, found him and saved his life. I have no memory of his face, or of his voice, or of his smell. All I know of him is what my mother told me. She said that he had a daughter who was a slave and that he wanted to free her. When he was healed from the snakebite, he and Mama walked for four days to Nashville where he joined the Federal Army so he could fight the slave owners.

After the battle, Mama said she looked for him for three days. She talked to the officers and men in his regiment who had survived; she walked back and forth over the battlefield and went to the hospitals. She went everywhere, but she never found him. Some of the gravediggers told her that he was probably in the big grave where they put a lot of the colored soldiers. She went there, but all she found was a muddy private's hat.

She never got over losing him. And, though I know she loved me, there were times I could see that her eyes were sad when she looked at me. I could see that she was far away and, though she never cried when this happened, I knew she was thinking about him. As I grew older she began to tell me about how she still missed my father and how, at times, when my face was turned a certain way and I was smiling, I looked like him.

Now, I am an old man with an old brain. When I was young, it seemed I could remember every detail of everything that I heard or saw. But now, there are times when I cannot remember what happened yesterday and sometimes not even this morning. Yet, and this is a wonder, I still remember people's faces and voices from long ago; I can still bring them up before me, just as they were when they were alive—smiling, laughing and crying, so real that sometimes I begin to smile or get tears in my eyes and I call them to me and hug them and kiss them.

As I write—sixty years later—about Mama and the Captain, I see her freckled face and Irish-red hair as clearly as I see my hand as I write, and I see the Captain and Lady, the Taggerts, Aunt Sally and Katey, our cabin on Elk River and the distant mountains; they are all here with me now. I hear their voices and Katey's barking, the sudden, loud splash of a fish, the calling of quail from the field beside the house, the strong smell of hickory wood burning, of rain, of newly turned earth and the sweet scent of honeysuckle. I feel the heat waves rising above the fields in mid-summer, the cool water of the river flowing slowly over me, and the touch of Mama's lips on my cheek at night after I've said my prayers.

Three months before the Captain died there was a full moon that was so large and bright it looked as though you could reach up and pull it from the sky. It was the last day of March, and the moon marked the time for us to plant our garden. The next morning Mama went to the shed behind the house and started getting the vegetable seeds ready and the other seeds, the ones she called her 'soul food'; for her flowers. I was on the porch whetstoning the hoes when Katey, our red feist, jumped from beside me and ran out into the yard, barking loudly. I stood and looked up the road.

Even at a distance, I could see the Captain coming down the road on Lady. His head and shoulders slumped forward like an old, sick man; his clothes hung on him like on a scarecrow. As he came closer, I could see his long beard and hair scraggling down from under a wide-brimmed straw hat. He rode slowly up to the edge of the yard and stopped. Now that he was close enough for Katey to smell him, she quit barking and came back to me, pressing her shoulder against my legs.

The mare climbed the bank from the road into the yard and walked up to the porch. The Captain looked more like a dead man than anyone I had ever seen who was still alive. His skin yellowish gray, his eyes sunk deep into their dark sockets. Hollowed cheekbones and protruding jawbones were almost covered by a white-streaked beard; long uncombed hair hung below his shoulders. His lips, colorless and thinned back tightly into a grimace; his hand's large bones and sinews and long, dirty fingers, with their broken nails, barely touched the reins that lay loosely curled across the pommel of the saddle. I could smell him.

Before the war, he had been a wealthy man. He had owned more than fifty slaves. Some had worked his fields, some he leased out. He had believed God favored slavery as a way to lift them out of darkness. He had had great pride in his thousand-acre plantation and in what he had achieved with his years of hard work. He had loved his family, Tennessee, and the South and had never doubted that their beliefs in honor, courage, and freedom would lead the South to victory. He had believed that God answered his prayers and would protect him and his sons in battle.

Now all of that was gone—all of it—but most of all his precious son was gone and he could not bear the pain that was inside him every day. He was alive and his son was dead. Even the love of his wife and the pleading of his two remaining sons and his friends and even with all the hugs and kisses of his six grandchildren, nothing that anyone did was enough. He turned more and more into himself and away from everyone else. And, as the years went by, his family gave up trying, and left him alone in his library with his books and his bourbon.

Three months after the war was over, he gave his bird dogs to Big Kinna who had served him faithfully for twenty years as the driver of his field hands and now lived alone in a cabin on the backside of the plantation. That Christmas the Captain quit going to church and began to eat alone. He seldom left the house. When night came, he fell asleep in the library, with his books and empty bottles scattered around him on the floor.

But now and then, on a Sunday evening, when there was no rain or heavy fog, he would hold back on his drinking just enough so he could walk without falling. An hour before sunset, he would put on his boots and tattered gray coat. Without a word to anyone, he would go out the back door, past the smokehouse, through the all-but-empty slave quarters, and down the slope to the pasture gate where he would whistle one time, high and clear. In an instant Lady would be there waiting for him as he unlatched and opened the gate, not closing it—for there were no other horses in the field—and walked through and on to the barn beyond with the mare so close behind him she was almost touching his shoulder with her head. At the barn, he led her into her stall and fed her a little grain while he groomed her coat and mane and tail until she stood glistening before him. Then he would talk to her about Bob. He would tell her what a beautiful little boy his son had been, how he tickled him at night before he went to sleep, how brave he was when he fell off his first pony and broke his arm and didn't cry, how handsome he was in his new uniform that last day at home, how he had shown no fear in all the fighting they had done; and how, when he died, he had not made the slightest sound as they fell together among the dead and wounded.

When he finished talking, he would bridle and saddle Lady, mount her, and ride off down the lane to the road where he would turn right and, a mile on, cross the river over Bethpage Bridge and then, for another mile, to a place where the road climbed to the top of Lynch Hill. There he would stop and stare at the mountains until the last light began to fade away, then he reined the horse around and rode back home in the dark. He told Mama all these things and I heard every word.

When Sunday evening came and the weather was good I would sit on the bank by the side of the road and wait for him to come by. Twice I hid in the woods beside the road and followed him all the way to Lynch Hill where I watched him from the shadows of the trees.

Even though he was dirty and skeletal and had once owned slaves, he was like a knight to me, a knight who had gone off to war to protect our land. I began to dream about him; and then, one night as I lay in bed, I began to pretend that he was my father and that he would teach me how to be like him, how to sit high up on a powerful war horse and how to fight, and when I was ready, he would take me with him into battle where I would be wounded and would ride home beside him with my empty sleeve pinned up just like his.

Yes, he had owned slaves and, yes, my father had been a slave; but it made no matter, for I was certain that the Captain loved me as he always nodded to me with a smile on his face and would say, "Good evening, Jeremiah," when he rode by on his way to Lynch Hill. And one evening, he lifted me up with his one arm onto the saddle in front of him and rode me to the bridge and back. I don't remember his saying a word until he brought me back and lifted me down, when he said, "Son, give my regards to your mother." That was the night I began to pretend he was my father. Now, I know it was just his way of talking.

Long years later, I went to Sewanee to talk with Aunt Sally about Mama and the Captain. She was in her eighties and blind when I visited her in her daughter's home. She was a little woman with tiny hands and feet; her skin was the color of dark chocolate. She puffed away on a small clay pipe as she told me about being the Taggerts' slave before the War; then staying on as their cook after it was over. She talked for an hour about Mama and the Captain and Miss Lucy; every now and then she would smile at a memory—but mostly her face was sad.

"Befo da wah, de Massah, he work hard, sometime he work in da field right long side of da hands. He hardly eva use tha whip on us, mostly he jus talk fuss talk when someone slackin. He sho luv Mistah Bob, he luv'd all his boys but Mistah Bob his favorite. Fo he change so, da Massah was a fun luvin man; but when he come home, he not da same man; all his smiles done lef im when dat boy died. I's think some of im done die right dere with Mistah Bob. Lawd, he done quit talkin, even to Miss Lucy, an he quit goin to da fields; he jus stay in dat room with dem ole books an all he did was drink dat bad stuff an eva now an den ride dat hoss of Mistah Bob's out to da Lawd knows where. He jus let his hair grow an be greasy an let 'isself get all smelly an not eat til he done shrink all away inside his skin.

"Lawd, Mistah Jeremiah, if it had'n been fo Miss Lucy makin 'erself into a man, we'd all died out dere for sure. She get up fo da ole roostuh dun crow an ring da bell an begin yellin fo da boys an da hands to get demselves up an out of bed an to da fields. She dun start cidin evathin; she say how much cotton, how much cawn, how much wheat dey goin to plant, an when to plant an when to pick. She make da sales an writ it all down in dem black books she keep in her room; she pick which mare to breed an which bull to buy; an many a day I seed her out dere in da fields sweatin with da hands an gettin all burn up by da sun til she turn black as me, an her flesh gettin so scratched by da stickuhs she look like she'd been whupped on like a runaway. An she keep all dis up an nevuh smile, til she start gettin hard, an her face start lookin like sum ole rock out in tha field.

"An Mistah Jeremiah, she get where she nevah show any hurt, but I know'd she be hurtin bout Mistah Bob dyin an den Mistah Robert same as dyin. But Miss Lucy she nevah show it, she done set her mind on holdin on to dat land an feedin her chullin an granchullin. But Mistah Jeremiah dere were times when dat chile was so bone tired she could'nt even go to sleep; an Mistah Jeremiah dere was sumpin else I seed, she didn't know I seed it but I did, sum nights when I heps her carry Mistah Robert to bed, I seed it in her eyes, how she be lookin at im, like she lookin at her own baby chile dat's dyin an ain't nothin she can do to stop it no mattuh how much she pray to da Lawd to not let im die, he jus keep dyin. I seed her unduh all dat hardness, dat po woman was still luvin Mistah Robert. It's da Lawd's truth Mistah Jeremiah, I done seed it all long ago in Miss Lucy, how dat da Lawd He put some good an some bad in all of us so's none of us be all good an none of us be all bad, an since we all His chullin He'll try to hep us all, even da bad ones to get ovuh da river to da othuh side to be with Him. Evuh since I know'd dat I's done lef most of da worryin to da Lawd when I's go's to sleep at night."

Aunt Sally was right, Lucy Taggert never stopped loving her husband. I know because I heard the Captain tell Mama about the nights his wife cried and cried and tried to love on him, and how he wouldn't let her, and how she begged him to do something to come alive again so he could love her and their family. I heard all of this, and I heard him say that it was Mrs. Taggert who got him to come ask my mother for help.

The sun was shining, but there was a nip in the air on that March morning when the Captain rode up to our house and looked down on me from Lady's back.

"Jeremiah, is your mother home?"

"Yes, sir."

"Would you please go and tell her that I would like to talk to her."

"Yes, sir."

I stepped off the porch and went around the side of the house to the backyard...stuck my head in the shed and told Mama that Captain Taggert wanted to talk to her. She said, "Tell him to have a seat on the porch and I'll be there in a minute. Did he say what he wants?"

"No'm," I answered.

When I came back to the front, the Captain had gotten down off of Lady and was standing by her with his hand on the pommel. He nodded but didn't move when I told him to come sit on the porch, that Mama was coming. I could see he didn't want to be there. He kept glancing over his shoulder, looking toward the road, as though he might see someone he knew might be passing by.

It seemed a long while until the front door opened and Mama stepped out onto the porch. "Good day to you, Captain Taggert." He took his hat off and nodded. "Can I help you?" she asked.

He began turning the hat around and around by the brim. At first he didn't look at Mama, he looked at the ground; then he looked again, over his shoulder, at the road and, seeing no one, turned back and looked at her. "Yes, um...uh, scuse me, could we talk private?"

Mama pointed to a post. "Tie your horse up and come inside," and walked back in the house leaving the door open. He moved slowly as he tied the reins to the post and climbed the steps and followed her inside and closed the door.

I ran back behind the house to the corncrib, pulled out an ear of corn, shucked some kernels into my hand, then ran back to Lady and began to feed her. Her eyes were large and beautiful; I could see myself reflected in them. For a moment, I felt almost as if I were being drawn into them; and then, from behind me, I heard the first low murmur of the Captain's voice inside the house, but I could not hear what he was saying.

My mother never knew that when people came to talk to her, that I hid under the window and listened to them telling her their secrets, telling sad things and, best of all, the bad things that they had done. It was exciting, though there were times when I heard something said that I wished I had not heard. Yet it never stopped me from listening.

I once asked Mama why people came to talk to her. We were sitting on the riverbank fishing. There was such a long moment before she answered that I thought she hadn't heard me, and then she said, "Well, Jeremiah, there's some people who keep all their bad feelings locked up inside until it builds up and begins to poison them; and after a while they're never happy and they start turning away from everybody, even the ones who loved them. Some get to drinking all the time, some stay angry all the time and think everybody's against them, some end up killing someone, some kill themselves. You know it's sorta like when you get risens coming up under your skin and I have to prick them with a hot needle to get the poison out. Well, that's what telling someone about the things hidden inside you can do, for some folks it lets out some of the angry things and the sad things, so, maybe, they can be a little happier."

When people came to talk to her she told me to stay outside, away from the house and not to make any noise. Of course. her not wanting me to hear what was being said made me want to hear every sound they made. So I was quiet as a mouse when I crawled on my belly down the side of the cabin until I was right under the window where I could hear every word and every whimper.

Lying there on my back, I heard people say some terrible things. To this day, I remember every word that was said by one of them—it has never left my ear; it was a man's voice that sounded almost like an animal, grunting and panting and talking all at the same time, it came from deep inside his throat as he told about burning alive a houseful of Negroes, "Unh, Unh, Unh...Oh God damn... I swear I didn't know those niggers had any children in there... Unh, Unh, Oh my dear God, I still hear them screaming, and I can still smell them...Oh God, what did I do?" and then, from deeper down, there came a long, guttural, groan, like a dying beast might make.

And I heard a woman say that she was dead, and I believed her, her voice was so empty and lifeless she did not sound human. She scared me. I thought that she was a ghost or a spirit, her voice in a faint whisper saying, "I died that first night. I was no longer alive. And after that I felt nothing, I heard nothing, I did not smell them as they put themselves in me, over and over, two white ones, two black ones and...white and black and white and black, over and over, and you know, all the time their faces were changing above me, sweating, biting their lips, touching fire to me, I saw the corn cob, I saw the light come and go into darkness and then the light and the dark returned...and there was something else...but it didn't matter for I was already dead the first night...nothing mattered...for I was dead."

I heard all kinds of things: sad, strange, scary, funny things, cruel things that people did to little children and old people and to prisoners and idiots, to each other and to animals. After awhile, I wondered where was God, why did He let these awful things happen, why didn't He just kill all the evil people. Then I began to worry that He would punish me for disobeying my mother. I was betraying her. But now, as I look back on it after all these years, I realize that if I had obeyed her, I wouldn't have learned how evil people can be, and how those who have been hurt badly or have done terrible things still keep on living, and how most of those who do awful things really want to be better than they are and that sometimes they do become better. How strange it is that I learned this from disobeying my mother. I know this though: If I had not hidden under that window I wouldn't have heard the Captain tell Mama about Bob.

So it was, on the first day the Captain came to our house and closed the door behind himself and began talking to Mama, that I threw down the corn that I was feeding Lady and crawled under the window just in time to hear the chair creak as he sat down and, in that same instant, I heard him begin telling Mama what had happened to Bob on June 4, 1864. The words poured out of his mouth without stopping, without emphasis, without life. It was only after awhile, when there was almost no more breath to say another word, that I heard his voice break.

"Sherman was Hell. He'd killed us all at Kennesaw if he'd had half a chance an that mornin he was goin to try again, he set on us hard with his cannons an when they stopped the air was so full of smoke an dust you could hardly breathe, you could taste the gunpowder an for a bit you could hardly see through all the smoke, the sun hangin like a drop of blood in the sky. The heat was terrible. It was over a hundred an there was no shade for we'd cut most of the trees down an what was left had been blown apart. As soon as the cannon stopped we began cleanin the dirt from our muskets an gettin ready for them. We knew they were comin. It was quiet now an everyone was whisperin so they wouldn't hear us behind that big wall of logs an dirt. Strange what you remember, way off there was a mule brayin over an over; the strangest thing, after all that noise an explosions, I heard a woodpecker hammerin away on a piece of wood just on the other side of the breastworks. isn't that strange that I'd remember it. My son was sittin by my side in the trench, he was leanin back against the mound with his eyes closed, his skin an beard were white with dust, his lips were so dry an cracked he looked old an worn an I wanted to touch him but I didn't. I let him sleep. Up an down the line I could hear the clinkin of ramrods an the clickin of hammers bein cocked an uncocked. It was still quiet but then from across the valley came the first sounds of their bugles. I shook Bob until he opened his eyes an sat up an he said somethin to me but I couldn't hear an he touched my hand, I leaned close to him an spoke in his ear, 'Stay by me, Bob, stay by me today;'

"I stood an looked over the top so I could see them an there they came seven long dark blue lines comin down the hill; the smoke had cleared an I could see their barrels an bayonets glistenin; I could see their battle flags an thousands of Yankees comin straight at us an everybody began to stand up to see them. We weren't afraid we knew how to kill, we were good at it, an then tough old Colonel Yeats shouted, 'Down, boys, down', an we knelt down without a sound an listened. We could hear the sound of their footsteps as they came closer an closer until they were so near we could hear their officers shoutin commands to their men who cheered louder an louder. The ground began to shake an then above it all. I heard that old Irishman's last call to us, 'Now, my precious boys, now, up an give em Hell,' an all of us rose up screamin an levelin our muskets at that mass of men who rushed towards us so near now we could see their faces. There was a great roar as we all fired together. I felt the heat like an oven on my face from the sheet of flame that burst outward from all along our breastworks sweepin away their first line. We fired an loaded, fired an loaded, slaughterin them in rows an heaps, killin them as fast as we could load an fire an still they came on stumblin an tramplin on their wounded an dead. Our cannons opened on them with canister. The air rushed an quivered; heads an arms were torn away; I saw half a body spinnin upward. They ran into our fire bent forward veerin away then back into the gaps firin as they came on an on right up to us. The air was filled with smoke an blood an the zippin an buzz of minie balls an their thuddin into flesh. Explosions an concussion were shakin the earth apart as we screamed an killed each other. I heard myself screamin, 'Kill em all! Kill em all!' an tasted sulfur an smelled shit an vomit an then it happened...there came a sound beside my head an with it a swash of wetness across my face an neck, an in that instant I was flung back an down hard on somethin an I saw before my eyes closed...I saw him...what had been my sweet boy...Oh Lord, Oh Lord...Goddamn God to Hell to burn with me forever for what He did that day to my dear boy who I did not save."

When he finished, there was a long silence; then I heard my mother, but she was talking so soft and low that I couldn't hear what she was saying. He stayed in the room with her for a good while, long enough that Lady and I both became restless; when I heard her begin pawing the ground, I crawled away from the window and went to her. Just as I was beginning to stroke her neck, the door opened and the Captain walked out, mounted and, without a word, rode away.

From that week on, on that same day, at the same hour, he returned. The third time he came they made love, and every time thereafter, for the next three months, they made love. I know they did. I heard it all, and I saw them six times through a hole that I made in the chinking between the logs. The last time he came, on June 27, 1874, he begged Mama to run away with him. When he said that, it scared me so I held my breath. There was a long silence, and then in a firm voice she said, "No, I'll not run away with you...I'm sorry, Robert, but I'll not do it, I don't love you...and I think it's best you stop coming here. I don't want to hurt you, but I don't think you should ever come back. It's best you go on home now."

He left.

That night he hanged himself.

A few nights later John Gaunt and the Taggerts came on horses. They were carrying torches. They hanged my mother high up in the big oak that grew beside the road in front of our cabin. They tried to find me but they couldn't; I was hiding deep in the cane on the bank of the river. The next morning when I got Mama's body down from the tree, I made my vow to kill them. And one winter day I did.

Even though I was a boy when all of this happened, and even though I loved my mother dearly, there was a long time when I believed that what she had done was wrong and that she was partly to blame for the Captain's death—it hurt me. But as I grew older and committed my own sins I began to think, who am I to stand in judgment of my mother who loved me so, who cared for me without anyone helping her, and who am I to judge anyone, even John Gaunt and the Taggerts, for I have done terrible things in my life: I have been a drunkard, and I have cursed God, I have been lascivious, and I have killed three people, so who am I to judge anyone?

NO COUNTRY FOR THE FEARFUL

Though some names have been changed this story happened as it is told. Only on occasions did I have to physically restrain someone. This is about one of those times when I was with a person who was paranoid and threatening others. I was never hurt, nor did I ever hurt anyone.

The phone rang.

I picked it up.

"Hello."

"Chief Holdan here, one of yours says she's gonna blow up tha bank."

"What's her name?"

"Her nephew says she's Gayle Clements an that she comes to see ya'll."

"Which bank?""

"Southern Farmers."

"Where's she now?"

"Outside on tha sidewalk. Thev've locked all tha doors."

"We're comin."

Five minutes later, Nancy Page, one of our staff who knew Clements, went with me downtown. We drove past the bank. A medium-sized woman was pacing back and forth on the sidewalk beside the bank. With quick, jerky, stiff-legged steps she looked up at the windows; the curtains were drawn tight, eyes peeked out between them.

It was 1978 in rural Tennessee. I was the third clinician hired for the new mental health clinic, having worked as a therapist at the Vanderbilt Child Psychiatric Hospital for eight years, and was a part-time employee for two summers in the Davidson County and Tennessee Psychiatric Hospitals in Nashville. I'd seen all kinds of mental illnesses. It had prepared me some for what was coming—but not entirely.

In those beginning years I had learned that people are not all good or all bad. Things had happened to them, bad genes, bad DNA, fetal injury; lots of things happen to us before we come out of the womb, and some right as we're coming out. Some of us cry our first outcry with good chemistry, some of us cry not so well, and then good things and bad things happen that bring to the surface the good and the bad.

In some ways it was the wild west; at times a barroom brawl. Four of us were serving eight counties, covering over four thousand square miles—more than two hundred thousand people. We saw any and everyone who came through the door, sometimes even out on the street, in jails, hospitals, wherever they were; people threatening to kill themselves or others, people seeing and hearing and believing in things that weren't there, alcoholics, abusers of every sort, members of the KKK, bestials, counseling schools with racial conflicts, delinquents, autistic children and adult people caught in the briers of life. Slowly we grew, adding more staff, then another county, a state prison.

It wasn't easy, at times it was hard, damn hard, at times scary but I can assure you it was never boring. There were even times when it was fun. I loved it and got so much more back than I gave. I had failures, but one thing I'm proud of: No one I personally cared for committed suicide or hurt anyone. And our center became, if not the best, a close second to best in Tennessee.

Well, let's get back to Mrs. Clements. We left her pacing back and forth looking up at the bank and, here and there, I could see eyes staring out of a slither of an opening in the curtains. I drove past and pulled into the parking lot in the back and went in the back door of the police station that was a short distance away across the lot.

Chief Holdan was waiting inside, with Mrs. Clements' nervous nephew who told us she had tried to kill her husband the night before but had the wrong size shotgun shells. To his knowledge she had no gun with her now though he didn't know about knives or dynamite.

Immediately we made our plan. The Chief called the county judge who agreed. I would approach Mrs. Clements first, backed up by two officers with Nancy behind them. I would try to get her to come with me voluntarily to the hospital. But if she refused and became agitated and threatening, the officers would come forward and help me restrain her, and then she would be taken by the officers to the hospital to see our psychiatrist who would evaluate her for commitment.

And that's pretty much the way it happened, except for one little glitch. I was only a few feet from her when she told me, "Go away!" and whirled around toward the open door of her car where I could see a large open handbag. As she reached in I grabbed her from behind and the officers came up quickly and handcuffed her and took her in a patrol car to the hospital.

In the bag was a large pair of shears.

WIND BIRD AND VICTOR

A Story of Two Wild Children

Though Wind Bird is not her actual name, a fair amount of this story is true, most especially her last wonderful words to me. Occasionally, I am asked, "What happened to her?" I don't know. I have never heard from her nor have I attempted to find her. In a way that is best for, as you will read, I have retained our magic and affection from those long years back where she remains ever young.

Scattered, fierce, and mute in earlier times,
Men wandered through the forests in all climes,
Clashing only with their fingernails for arms
They filled the woods with death cries and alarms,
The state of these our savage forebears in the wild,
We see before us in this young child.

—Louise Racine

The wild child may have been a reassuring witness that, no matter how utterly a child is rejected by its parents, there is a benign nature that looks after all its children. The ubiquity and timelessness of such speculations cannot be doubted.

—Harlan Lane
The Wild Boy of Aveyron

We will always carry each other around in our hearts forever.

—Wind Bird

So I have carried you in my heart all these fifty plus years; even now, at seventy-nine, I see you standing in the open doorway of my office in your canary-yellow dress, your eyes and hair black as crow's wings, your skin dark honey. You say these words, turn away into the hallway and are gone—forever.

She was wild. Not feral. Not autistic. Not retarded. Wild. Unpredictable. Sometimes making animal sounds. She was short and strong, at times dangerous. Her mother, full blood Cherokee. Father unknown. She was eleven when she came all those hundreds of miles from Wears Valley, from the foothills of the Smokies, to the Vanderbilt Children's Psychiatric Unit in Nashville.

Three days after her arrival, she leapt onto an attendant's back, grabbing him around his neck, pulling him backwards, twisting him to the floor, all the while grunting deep in her throat. The third week, she tripped a nurse with a broom handle, spraining her wrist. The fourth week she disappeared. The doors to the ward were locked. No one saw her run out. In an instant she had disappeared. Searching, and looking and looking; she was not there.

And then, a tiny, mouse-like, eight-year-old boy, a tiny, fair-skinned boy, who had smothered his baby sister to death, pointed to a corner pillar, jutting out from the wall where a low wooden cabinet was built against the pillar. We got down on our knees, opened the cabinet door and saw an opening into the pillar. She was there just above us, just a bit inside the pillar,

She came out, kicking, scratching, and growling.

❖

Born in freezing winter, the girl-baby came quickly out of her squatting mother onto a cold, dirty gunnysack that lay on the dirt floor of a tarpaper shack at the bottom of a steep-sided hollow. The mother tied a leather shoestring around the cord and cut the cord with a dull knife while the baby lay screaching. The mother grimaced. She looked down at the wet, flailing baby, "I'll be damn, she's gotta lotta wind in er...I think I'm gonna call er, Wind."

An old man watched all of this with his watery, half-shut eyes. He was sitting in a ladder-back chair beside a tilted iron pot-bellied stove that was growing cold. He barely nodded through his blurred vision, then drank a long swallow from the fruit jar always beside him; his eyelids flickered; his shoulders slumped and he slept.

"Goddamnit, Daddy, hit's freezin in yair, git up an git some wood an git tha far a-goin. I need ta heat up some water an clean that little un an myself." The old man didn't open his eyes or move. She picked up a piece of kindling, threw it and hit his knee. "You'uns go git some wood an build this far back up."

"Damn! That, done hurt like hell!" He rubbed his knee for a moment then staggered to his feet and out the door. Even through the log wall he could hear the screeching of the baby.

Among the many men who came to her, Wind's mother had no idea who the father was, for they never seemed to stop coming down the steep, narrow footpath that led from the ridge road. Down and up the hill they came and went, Indians and whites and even an occasional black man; most brought money, some whiskey, a few came with chickens or a shoat.

And year after year, as she grew older, more and more, her mother would send Wind out of the house when the men came. But there were times, if the weather was bad, when she was kept inside. Then, she would curl herself into a ball under a filthy scrap of blanket in the corner farthest from the only bed in the room. With her fingers in her ears she tried not to breathe she was so frightened of her mother and the man. It was then that she began to run away into her mind, disappearing into the woods, listening to the animals and birds panting and groaning and crying and calling to her.

While most of the men paid no attention to her, a few spoke kindly, but there was one who pulled the blanket off and began to fondle her until her mother broke a crock jar on his back and threatened to cut his throat. Her grandfather did nothing but drink and sleep, and stare into the fire until his daughter threw something at him. Then, he would stagger out and cut more wood or bring a bucket of water from the spring.

She was eight the first time she ran away into the woods and stayed gone for three days and nights until hunger and the cold drove her back to the cabin. But, as time went on, she ran away again and again. And, as she grew older, she stayed away longer and longer, eating wild plants, fruits, nuts, roots; sleeping in the hollows of trees; speaking to animals.

She told me these things. She drew them on paper. She made their sounds and drew pictures of the animals and of herself with them. Slowly, she taught me to understand.

I began to read about feral and wild children. Most especially, I was taken by a small book by Jean-Marc-Gaspard Itard, French physician and educator of the deaf. Published in 1801 his, *An Historical Account of the Discovery and Education of a Savage Man, or of The First Developments of the Young Savage Caught in The Woods Near Aveyron, In The Year 1798.* Victor, the "Wild Boy of Aveyron", was brought to the National Institute for the Deaf in 1800. There he met Itard who affectively adopted Victor and began to attempt to teach him to speak and communicate with others and "to develop him physically and morally".

A child of eleven or twelve, who some years before had been seen completely naked in the Caune Woods seeking acorns and roots to eat, was met in the same place toward the end of September 1799 by three sportsmen who seized him as he was climbing into a tree to escape their pursuit. Conducted to a neighboring hamlet and confined to the care of a widow, he broke loose at the end of a week and gained the mountains, where he wandered during the most rigorous winter weather, draped rather than covered with a tattered shirt. At night he retired to solitary places but during the day he approached the neighborhood villages where of his own accord he entered an inhabited house...

Jean-Marc-Gaspard Itard

A small bit of me was as she was—Cherokee—my father's father, olive-skinned, high, rounded cheekbones, great, great, grandson of James Vann, leader of the Upper Villages; hunter, whiskey maker, lover of wild things. So my father. So am I.

I was drawn to her—to our shared blood.

She came all those many hundreds of miles from the mountains of East Tennessee to Nashville without family, without a friend, with only a social worker who did not know her, a woman whose eyes were scared, whose eyes said, 'I want to get this over with and go home,' who, as soon as she put the records on my desk and signed the admission papers, fled without a glance or a word of goodbye to Wind. As the door of the ward closed behind her there was nothing in Wind's eyes. I put my hand on her shoulder and she jerked away.

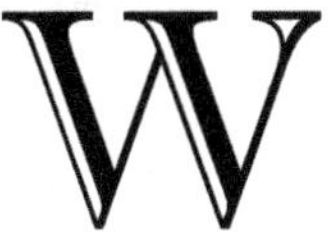ind Bird's records were in two tattered, gray folders; together, they were three inches thick. I opened the first one and began to read:

Referring Provider: Smoky Mountain Mental Health Center

Date: May 10, 1966

Patient: Wind Bird. **Age**: 11. **Born**: July 7, 1954. **Place of Birth**: At home in: Wears Valley, Tennessee. **Parents: Father**: Unknown **Mother**: Storm Bird, full blood Cherokee. **Education**: Possibly, Grade 2. **Religion**: Unknown. **Race**: Cherokee. **Health History**: Old scars are on her legs, arms and hands; otherwise, no health problems. Though there are times she will not communicate her hearing, speech, and vision are unimpaired. After removal from her home in March she was taken to the Sevier County Public Health Department for physical examination, at which time she received all immunizations.

Behavior History: From early childhood patient has had serious behavior problems in the home, school, and community. Becomes angry at the slightest provocation, during which she may scratch, bite, or strike others. She has destroyed eggs of setting hens, pulled blossoms from fruit trees, opened gates and let livestock out, poured the contents of slop-jars into cisterns, and prevented postmen from continuing their route by refusing to move from in front of their car. She has been dismissed from school five times for fighting classmates, teachers, and school bus drivers. When enraged, she makes guttural and screeching sounds like animals. But, by far the most potentially dangerous behaviors for herself are her frequent runaways into the forest, where bear, wild boar, and poisonous snakes abound. She may stay gone for several days and nights, twice for more than a week. During this time she lives off of wild plants, nuts, and fruits and vegetables that she steals from gardens. At the time of her removal her mother no longer notified the authorities but allowed her to remain gone until she returned home.

Removal From Home: As a result of complaints from school authorities and members of the community the patient was removed from her home by the

Sevier County Public Welfare Department on March 1, 1966 and placed in a Child Detention Home. Subsequently, by order of Sevier County Juvenile Judge Jack Stanley the Mental Health Center saw the patient twice: March 14 and April 12.

Evaluation: Though the patient was resistant to testing and interviewing she is in no way psychotic, intellectually limited, deaf, mute or autistic. Rather, she appears to be highly observant and reactive to others in a manner that suggests her driving force is to avoid being controlled by others and, failing this, her aggressive impulses are to combat them and, that failing, to flee from them.

Due to the abuses she has experienced, it might well be surmised that beneath her aggressive behavior is a great amount of fear and need for security, acceptance, and affection.

It is our belief that this patient will benefit from a period of hospitalization followed by prolonged residential care during which time she should receive schooling and regular psychotherapy. Her mother is agreeable with this recommendation and does not oppose the Tennessee Department of Public Welfare having custody of her daughter.

Payment: Payment for the patient's hospitalization will be made by the Tennessee Department of Mental Illness and Mental Retardation.

[The boy was] a disgustingly dirty child affected with spasmodic movements, and often convulsions, who swayed back and forth ceaselessly like certain animals in a zoo, who bit and scratched those who opposed him, who showed no affection for those who took care of him; and who was, in short, indifferent to everything and attentive to nothing.

[Escape was his obsession,] when observed in his room...his eyes [turned] constantly toward the window, gazing sadly into space. If a stormy wind then chanced to blow, if the sun suddenly came from behind the clouds brilliantly illuminating the skies, he expressed an almost convulsive joy with clamorous peals of laughter, during which all his movements backward and forward very much resembled a kind of leap he would like to take, in order to break through the window and dash into the garden. Sometimes instead of these joyful emotions, he exhibited a kind of frantic rage, wrung his hands, pressed closed fists to his eyes, gnashed his teeth audibly, and became dangerous to those who were near him.

I was Wind's therapist. I saw her twice a week in my office during the year she was in the hospital, and afterwards once a week during the three years she was in the Christian Children's Home in Nashville.

I was never afraid of her. She never attacked me. At the beginning, I was intellectually fascinated by her being Cherokee and by her past life and behavior, then over time I began to like her, and toward the end we came to love one another. She was special.

At first, she did not want to come. But when she understood we would leave the ward she came readily. I knew she saw this as a chance to escape. My hand stayed near her. She knew it. So she never lunged away. She said nothing. She walked beside me down the hallway and turned into my office. I closed the door behind us. So we began.

That first time, for twenty minutes or so, she roamed around the office carefully studying photographs and pictures on the walls, most especially the etchings of a gyrfalcon and a red-tailed hawk. I could see her eyes fix on the hawk's eyes; slowly she raised her right arm, reached out with her fingers and gently stroked the hawk's head as she made faint, high-pitched sucking sounds between her closed lips. She turned and looked at me. There was no expression on her face. "I help hawks that have been hurt. I'm a falconer," I said.

She continued around the office now and then picking up objects and smelling them, once putting a small bronze deer to her mouth and touching it with the tip of her tongue. From across my desk, she saw a green vase filled with hawk feathers. She could not reach the vase from her side so she came around until she was by my chair. She took three feathers out and rubbed them across her face, again making sucking sounds.

The office had a large window. The blinds were raised. It looked out into a manicured, grassy courtyard with two large oaks. The air was green with the sun's brightness. She stood in front of the window; for a long while she stared at the grass and trees and sky. And then, suddenly, she sprang upward onto the windowsill and began to pound with her fists on the glass panes, making little sounds and crying, "Please...Please...Please!" until I grabbed her around the waist and pulled her down. She growled, and kicked , and scratched, and cursed.

[These are my aims:]

1st To interest [the wild boy] in social life by rendering it more pleasant for him than the one he was then leading, and above all more like the life he had just left.

2nd To awaken his nervous sensibility by the most energetic stimulation, and occasionally by intense emotion.

3rd To extend the range of his ideas by giving him new needs and by increasing his social contacts.

4th To lead him to the use of speech by subjecting him to the necessity of imitation.

5th To make him exercise the simplest mental operations, first concerning objects of his physical needs and later the objects of instruction.

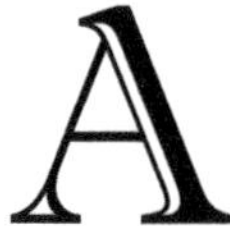ll I sought at first was her trust.

The next day, I gave her a red-tailed hawk's tail feather.

She took it and turned away.

The next day she was waiting at the door in the ward.

That day, in my office, she drew a picture filled with trees and birds and animals. They were highly detailed and realistic. Above them was something that resembled a face, part animal, part human. She would not tell me what it was or explain what it meant. She handed the picture to me. I thanked her. She said nothing. She made no sounds.

The next day, when I unlocked the door, and stepped inside, she was hunkered down next to the wall; she looked up at me, straight into my eyes. Without a word she stood up and took my hand. When we entered my office she immediately saw her picture taped to the wall next to my desk. Her mouth opened slightly as though she were about to speak. But she did not. From that day on she was always waiting at the door when I came.

I learned from the head nurse that she loved fruits and nuts and raw eggs, so I began to keep them in my office as treats. Slowly she began to make quick smiles and talk with me in her mountain language.

Then, three months along, I knew Wind trusted me as I trusted her. I began to take her out of the building onto the grounds. And it was that first day, as we went out into the courtyard, I saw her cry. Then she dried her eyes, looked straight into the sun and smiled and began to whistle like a quail.

As the months passed, our walks lengthened taking us beyond the courtyard to the larger campus with its wide yards, trimmed hedges, oaks, maples, magnolias, and elms. Whether a burning hot day or a freezing cold one, she had the habit, as we left the building, of stopping and raising her face to the sky with her mouth opened wide and flicking her tongue out to, "taste tha ire, fer hit feeds me." And then, she would run ahead: skipping, leaping, twirling, whistling, cawing, chirping and, now and then, when she came to her special maple with its low limbs, she would spring up onto it's trunk and climb fast as a squirrel and scoot out onto a limb from where she would gesture for me to join her, laughing, "Mr. Spain, yer a big ole sissy."

How could I not love her?

[Once in an attempt to teach Victor vowel sounds Itard rapped Victor's fingers with a small stick when he erred in the task.] *I cannot describe how unhappy he looked*

with his eyes thus closed and with tears escaping from them every now and then. Oh! How ready I was on this occasion, as on many others, to give up my self-imposed task and regard as wasted the time I had already given to it! How many times did I regret ever having known this child, and freely condemn the sterile and inhuman curiosity of the men who first tore him from his innocent and happy life...

[And later, as his despair for Victor making any significant improvement increased, Itard wrote,] *Unhappy creature, I cried as if he could hear me, and with real anguish of heart...since my labors are wasted and yours fruitless, take again the road to your forests and the taste for your primitive life. Or if your new needs make you depend on a society in which you have no place, go, expiate your misfortune, die of misery and boredom at Bicetre [the asylum]*

Wind lived in the hospital for a year. Gradually, outwardly, she became domesticated. Her outbursts of rage became fewer and fewer, her attacks on others stopped; she no longer attempted to flee. She began to read and write and sit at a desk, to use a knife and fork instead of her hands; most special to me, she began to laugh at funny things and look sad when she heard something that was sad. Yet, she still did not participate in games and play with the other children. Other than me and a motherly nurse and a young woman teacher, she showed little feeling toward the other adults and often scowled at them when she was told to do something she did not like.

It was only when I received permission to take her and two other children, and an aide, off the ward to a remote lake within a hilly forest that stretched for miles and miles did I see that the wildness was still in her. For, as soon as we were out of the car, she ran ahead making her animal sounds and leapt into the lake and swam out, dipping under water, then springing up and shouting, "Come on...come on...come on!" And I did. And we did. And it was at that moment, as if she was my daughter.

When the severity of the season drove every other person out of the garden, he delighted in taking many turns around it; after which he used to seat himself on the edge of a basin of water. I have often stopped for whole hours together, and with unspeakable pleasure, to examine him in this situation; to observe as all of his convulsive motions, and that continual balancing of his whole body diminished, and by degrees subsided to give place to a more tranquil attitude and how insensibly his face, insignificant or distorted as it might be, took the well-defined character of sorrow, or melancholy reverie, in proportion as his eyes were steadily fixed on the surface of the water, and when he threw into it, from time to time, some remains of withered leaves. When in a moonlight, the rays of that luminary

penetrated into his room he seldom failed to awake out of his sleep, and to place himself before the window. There he remained, during a part of the night, staring motionless, his neck extended, his eyes fixed towards the country illuminated by the moon, and, carried away in a sort of contemplative ecstasy, the silence of which was only interrupted by deep-drawn-inspirations, after considerable intervals, and which were always accompanied by a feeble and plaintive sound.

A few days after her twelfth birthday Wind was discharged to a Christian Children's Home in Nashville. I continued to see her twice a month for three years. With patience, love and firmness her house parents and teachers transformed her into a well spoken, courteous, and considerate person. And, with their help, she reached her appropriate grade level in school in two and a half years. How we celebrated! I gave her copies of the Audubon Field Guide to the Southeastern States and a collection of Wordsworth's poetry. Not only had she caught up in school but her pronunciation was, but for an occasional lapse, free of mountain dialect.

On July 7, 1970, Wind's fifteenth birthday, I received the phone call I knew would one day come. She was returning home. Her mother, Storm Bird, had reformed her own life. She was no longer a prostitute. She had stopped drinking and joined the Wears Valley Pentecostal Church. Her father was dead. She had a full-time job as a housekeeper at a resort hotel at the edge of the Park. She had moved into the small town and rented a house trailer. She wanted her daughter back. After verifying the mother's stability to properly care for Wind, the Home's social worker was taking her home.

I saw her the last time on July 14, 1970. We held hands walking across the campus; neither of us spoke. She stopped before her favorite climbing tree, let go of my hand, walked over to the tree, reached around the trunk, pressed her cheek against it and hugged it.

We returned to my office where we both cried. Then the time came, she turned away into the hallway and was gone forever.

Later on, months later, I attempted to contact her. I was not successful. I never heard from Wind again.

We will always carry each other around in our hearts forever.

Finally, however, seeing that the continuation of my efforts and the passing of time brought about no change, I resigned my efforts to the necessity of giving up any attempts to produce speech, and abandoned my pupil to incurable dumbness...I was obliged to restrain myself

and once more to see with resignation [my] hopes, like so many others, vanish before an unforeseen obstacle.

In 1828, Victor died in the home of Madame Guerin, his caretaker. He was forty. Itard died ten years later.

❖

Dear Wind,

Are you still alive? Did you marry? Did you have children? How are you? I pray that you are well and that you are happy. You are still in my heart. Am I in yours?

Love,
George Spain
January 2016

LAFE

Lafe is an entirely fictional character living in Lost Cove, a real valley a few miles south of the University of the South, Sewanee, Tennessee. Today, he would likely be diagnosed as having schizophrenia. He was created to see what might happen if placed against my hero, Jeremiah.

Lafayette Washington Pearson
1860–1878

Once't, when I wus born, I wus two people, Angel an Lafe together, all at tha same time, an somehow or other Angel weren't right, she could nair walk, nair talk, nair care fer herself, but I loved her dearly anyways since she wus me; so I went up in tha barn loft an prayed ta God ta make her right, an I cuts my arms an bled all over ta shed blood fer her, an I ask im that made us ta make us over agin, but He didn't do nuthin, we jus stayed like we wus; so's I became jes Lafe by myself, an I stays away in tha woods from Angel an Nanny an tha other'ns, much as I could; but all that happened a long while later, a long while after tha giant came on me on his big black horse outta tha trees; an when I think on hit, I still hyair his voice an smell im an see im killin my dog, Queenie, an then killin Daddy an Brother.

Nanny

Fer a long bit hit wair a mystery ta me, why neither of tha twins wair made right; they'uns jes weren't natural, they wair not hardly like human beins from tha first when they'uns come outa me, cept maybe Lafe he'uns seemed normal until what happened ta im, but you'uns could see Angel weren't. I studied on hit fer a long while an then I prayed on hit fer a long while an then, one day hit come ta me that hit wair a punishment brought down on me fer my ways with tha Garner boys, a long way back when I wus only a youngun an had nairy a bit of sense. But I guess from tha Lord's way uv lookin at hit I wus sinnin an had ta pay tha price. But hit don't seem rite that Angel an Lafe had ta suffer fer my sins; tha Lord should uv jes done sumpin ta me an be done with hit but, no, them pore thangs, specially Lafe, lived most in misery; but thair's somethin good an different inside Angel that sumtimes I think's maybe like a real angel, I seed hit, fer she'uns wus always happy, even tho she can't tell hit ta us in words. Oh, dair God, fergive me fer bringin tha sufferin on her.

Jeremiah

The first time I saw him; he was coming straight toward me down a long field through the first soft-gray light of evening. He looked like a young Viking: slender and fair with long blonde hair spread across his shoulders; his face as pretty as a girl's, with full lips and long eyelashes; his movements smooth as water; his eyes pale, unblinking, cold and hard, the eyes of a killer. He wore patched dove-gray pants, no shirt and an unbuttoned, threadbare blue cavalry jacket and no shoes. In the crook of his right arm was a double-barreled shotgun, stuck in his pants was a Colt pistol, a long skinning knife was sheathed in a scabbard attached to a wide leather belt around his waist. He had two large brindle hounds with him, one on each side. He was fourteen.

Lafe

I wus four, when hit all happen. I still see hit an hyair hit...Queenie smelt em first; she set ta barkin, an runnin back an forth right side me in tha wagon, an when she seed all em horsemen a comin outa tha woods, she went ta growlin. They'uns so quiet at first, Daddy an Brother didn't see or hyair em, fer they're choppin on tha farwood but then tha horsemen rode up all round us an they stopped choppin. One of em was a giant. He wus on a big black horse an he come right up side tha wagon, right next ta me an I commenced ta shiverin he look so much like a big bear ridin on a horse. I could barely see his eyes when they'uns look down at me through all that hair an beard coverin his face over. He skeered me so I pretended ta be daid an hoped he'd think so to, an go away. But he nairy went. He reach down an grabbed a hold uv me an hitched me up an spread-legged me round his neck so's I wus facin toward Daddy an Brother. All tha other horsemen had gotten down off their horses an were standin all round em; an when I see'd my Daddy I didn't call ta im or cry cause I wus daid.

Nairy a one hep me, not even God, maybe He wus daid too, fer thair come a time way later on, when I knowed He'd died too. Tha giant's hair stank an, got grease on me an, I wus hurtin twixt my legs where I'd been pull't down hard. Two men, jest alikes, were beatin on Daddy an Brother while tha other'uns held em; then they started a cuttin on em an Daddy was cussin an Brother nastied hisself. Queenie jumped from tha wagon through tha air an grabbed hold of tha giant's arm an bit im an he took hold of her an twisted her head an pitched her ta tha ground, an she nair moved agin. An I member tha mule's eyes gettin all big but thair bodies nair moved or made a sound, they'uns pretendin they'uns daid too. Then tha giant, he lifted me round in front of im an kiss me full on tha mouth an set me easy back in tha wagon an shouted at tha look alikes ta get thair hair an finish hit all up. Though my eyes be daid they seen Daddy an Brother's skin an hair cut off thair heads an tha jest alikes tied tha hair ta tha reins uv tha giant's horse an they'uns put ropes round Daddy an Brother's necks an haul'd em way high up in a tree, then they'uns all rode off. But I jest stayed daid fer apiece til Nanny an tha girls come. An when they seed hit all thair eyes got scairt lookin at what wair up in tha tree but I weren't scairt cause I wus daid an I hain't aire been scairt agin.

Lillie Jane

Lafe was killed when I had just turned four so I barely remember him. What little I do remember is mostly sad and unpleasant, the fact be known, he sometimes scared me. One time, I heard him in the kitchen with Angel - they were alone—he was talking to her like they were having a conversation; he'd make moaning sounds just like she did, as though she was talking back to him. It made me run and hide. He was different than anyone I've ever known, different, more than even Angel. There were two things that "marked him", as Nanny used to say about terrible happenings and what they could do to children: the first must have been a horror, for he was only four when he saw Daddy and Brother being killed right in front of him; then they were scalped and skinned; my Lord, that's beyond my imagining. The second was Angel's deformity; Nanny told me how he tried to get God to make her right. He cut his arms until they were covered in blood. When Angel was not changed into a perfect girl, Lafe turned his back on God, even on us; he stayed to himself, sleeping for days out in the woods, hunting and killing animals; coming to the house for only a day or so and then he was gone again.

Jeremiah

Lafe has never left me. How could this strange boy have been my wife's brother? It was as if he and Lillie Jane came from different parents: he fair, somber, easy to anger, with the language of the mountains; she dark, smiling, filled with laughter and color whose speech is of one well-educated.

When I was with him I was careful with my words and movements. He could be abrupt and would flair up if anyone, even his mother, opposed him. Yet with all of this, I was awed by his independence, his brilliance in the wild and his harsh honesty; the more we were together, the more I wanted to be like him.

When we were in the woods, if he sensed the presence of an animal or a human, he would throw up his arm for me to stop. Except for the flaring of his nostrils he would stand still as a stone; his whole being would be fixed on whatever he saw or heard or felt was nearby. His eyes darted back and forth; he sniffed the air like an animal; the tip of his tongue would flick out and twitch as he tasted the air. If it had been possible, his ears would have twisted and turned like a deer's.

Though I know it is foolish, it has gone through my mind that he wasn't quite human; yet I never thought he was insane or possessed. The old woman, Maw-ree, who lived in a cave on the side of the mountain, who some called a witch was with me when I first saw Lafe coming up the field; she said, 'Dat un comin der be a debil.' No, that is not right, she was wrong, for though he was different than anyone I've ever known, Lafe was not a devil. Within him, I could see the little boy loving his father and brother who were slaughtered before his eyes, and I could see the brother whose heart was broken as he heard his sister, twisted in her crib, moaning over and over. How can such terror and sadness ever be known by any of us?

Nanny

After he seen Nathaniel an James kilt by John Gaunt an his trash Lafe turned different an thair weren't a bit of joy left in im. An after he cut hisself all up fer Angel an hit nairy changed her, that's when tha demon got in im an from then on he acted like he ain't got no more carin fer anyone. He quit lookin at Angel an if we'uns go ta tech im, he'd pull away. He even made a fist at me onct an had a look in his eye like he'd hit me if I laid a hand on im. He'd usually jest grunt or look away if ya said airy a thang to im. His eyes'd git all dead lookin an at night when he wus in tha loft, he'd laugh an holler an shout blackguards an thair's times he'd growl an his voice'd go deep inside im like he wus someone else.

All those last yairs, fore he wus kilt, he'd hardly hit a lick ta hep us with tha stock or crops. Tha biggest part uv his time wus spent with his dogs an guns back in tha woods an on tha mountin; when he'd kill somethin he bloodied his face an put tha meat on tha table an ud start actin out how he'd kilt hit an cut hit's throat; an he'd git ta makin tha gun sounds an tha dyin sounds. His eyes'd be all big an shiny til he stopped then they'd go daid agin an he'd go up ta tha loft an fall asleep. Lookin back on hit all, hit aire a great sadness—fer he wair my baby boy...my baby boy.

Lafe

Tha Cove's full uv spirits, specially in tha cave or mongst tha beeches whair tha Injuns worshipped. Tha spirits nairy trouble me fer I leave em offerins on tha oak tree atop tha cliff above tha Sink.

Jeremiah

"Shit, yer still a kid an don't know nairy bout killin but by God I'll turn ya inta a killer. We'll kill that sumbitch Sheriff an tha otherns." That's what Lafe promised me. The next morning he took me into the woods above the Sink to a tree where he had hung carcasses, skulls, skins of animals and feathers of birds. While I watched, he circled the tree chanting over and over, " Tutsihusi Tutsihusi Tutsihusi," a Cherokee word that meant, "Die Die Die."

I killed my first deer, a doe, a week later. As we knelt beside her Lafe put both of his hands on her body, closed his eyes and said something that sounded like another language, then pulled his knife from its scabbard, cut her throat and let the blood flow over his hands. He lifted them, turned to me and rubbed the blood over my face and in my hair. "Now, ye be baptized in tha name of tha one who loves killers." With that, he sliced her stomach open, reached inside, cut her heart out and handed it to me. "Eat hit! Eat ever speck uv hit!"

Three years later, when I was fourteen and he eighteen, we killed a giant she-bear, the last bear killed in Lost Cove. She killed two of our dogs and nearly killed Lafe. When he shot her, she charged and fell on him. I thought he was dead. Just as she was about to bite him I shot her in the eye and finished her. It was quiet for a minute then, I heard laughter and Lafe rolled out from under her, covered in blood, "Jeremiah yer ready, hits time fer us ta kill that sumbitch Sheriff an em other sumbitches!"

Lafe

God let Angel die but I didn't cause I kept her alive all inside me whair we'uns talk all tha time, most at night, an she'uns ull tell me she loves me an I tell her I love her. But sometimes we'uns git ta arguing, specially bout me likin ta kill things, but I tells her I can't hep hit fer hit takes some uv tha hurt in me away fer a bit. Fer I still see Daddy an Brother daid up in em trees all tha time, an I git so scairt hit drives me ta want ta kill tha giant an his'uns. So I tells Angel ta stop fussin at me cause I got ta git ready fer killin em; so I keep on killin wild things an Angel keeps on fussin though I know she still loves me cause I can see hit in her face an she can still see hit in mine....

Lillie Jane

On December 22, 1878, my brother, Lafayette Washington Pearson, and Jeremiah Vann killed Sheriff John Gaunt, his sister Lucy Taggert and her twin sons, Sam and Hubert Taggert, on the road between Sewanee and Sherwood. Lafe was killed by John Gaunt. The next day, we buried him beside Daddy and Brother in the Pearson cemetery in Lost Cove.

Nanny

Losin yair babies might nigh kills ya; hit nair leaves ya; tha hurtin's waitin thair ever mornin rite side yair bed.

PART THREE

WORDS FOR POLITICIANS AND OTHERS

Following are speeches and presentations given to State Legislators, advocacy organizations, board members, and families; newspaper articles; letters to editors, colleagues and others; and a variety of reports and commentary. These copies of the originals are organized chronologically from the late 1960s to the beginning of 2000. They reflect my thoughts, beliefs and actions in real time as events were unfolding.

MENTAL ILLNESS HISTORY FRAGMENTS

The following historical fragments chronicle the treatment of people with mental illness. It is a story of many well meaning failures, some cruelties and some triumphs. It recounts our continuing search to understand what causes these illnesses and how to treat them. This history should warn us of the unintended and sometimes tragic consequences hidden within the progress and beliefs of the moment. It should also inspire us to never give up until all mental illnesses are eliminated. Now, we are at the dawning of the Human Genome, a time of great hope -- and of potential danger if the knowledge gained is misused.

"O that way madness lies; let me shun that; no more of that."

-- King Lear
Act III: Scene IV,
1608

1000 B.C. I Samuel 21:10-15	David "changed his behavior before them, and feigned himself mad in their hands, and he scrabbled on the doors of the gate, and let his spittle fall down upon his beard."
50 – 60 A.D. Mark 5:1-17	Jesus encounters "a man with an unclean spirit . . . neither could any man tame him." Jesus casts the spirits out into a herd of swine and the man was "in his right mind."
130 – 200 AD	Galen, a Roman physician, states that mental disorders are due to an excess in black bile, necessitating bleeding and purgatives.
1300 -- 1600	In Europe, tens (possibly hundreds) of thousands of people are convicted of demon possession and witchcraft and are tortured and executed. It is believed that some were mentally ill.
1692	Salem Witch Trials are held in Massachusetts. Twenty people are convicted of witchcraft. Nineteen are hung and one is pressed to death.
1751	Quakers and Benjamin Franklin establish the first hospital in America (Pennsylvania) for the "lunatics . . . distempered in mind and deprived of their rational faculties. . ." Lunatic is a word now outdated, but long used for people with mental illness, based on a belief that lunacy fluctuated with phases of the moon.
1792	Philippe Pinel, French physician, unchains fifty "maniacs" in Paris hospital and originates use of "moral treatment."
1796	English Quakers found the Retreat in York where they expand use of Pinel's moral treatment in the belief that in a healthy, structured, active, kind, and moral environment the patient's mind will be redirected and comforted.
1796	Tennessee becomes a state. Pauper lunatics let out to lowest bidder for one year term. Violent lunatics confined in jails, others in poor houses.
1831	146 Maury County, Tennesseans petition the State legislature to use part of the new penitentiary "as a sort of hospital" with regular physician care and safe keeping of lunatics.

1832	Tennessee's legislature authorizes $10,000 to build a hospital for 200 persons.
1840	Lunatic Asylum of Tennessee opens, the eleventh institution for the mentally ill in the United States. Built on a rise not far from present Union Station in Nashville. First two patients are pauper men from Lincoln County.
1842	Green Grimes, from Maury County, Tennessee is admitted to the Asylum in June. Writes: A SECRET WORTH KNOWING and A LILY OF THE WEST for physicians and families to better understand needs of the insane.
1847	Dorothea Dix, United States' greatest advocate for the mentally ill, comes to Tennessee and sends to the Tennessee General Assembly a "Memorial, Soliciting Enlarged and Improved Accommodations for the Insane of the State of Tennessee by the Establishment of a New Hospital." She finds that the existing hospital's conditions are deplorable.
1852	New hospital, Tennessee Hospital for the Insane, with 138 rooms and 250 acres opens on Murfreesboro Road near Nashville. This hospital's name is later changed to Central State. (The original 1840 hospital is used for wounded in Civil War. It burns down before the war ends).
1861-65	Nashville is occupied by Federal army which stations troops and horses on hospital grounds. Physicians and staff continue to care for patients even though they receive no pay.
1868	The Ewing Building, the first hospital in United States for insane blacks, opened on property of the Tennessee Hospital for the Insane.
1886	East Tennessee Hospital for the Insane opened in Knoxville.
1889	West Tennessee Hospital opened in Bolivar.
1890-1960	Moral treatment does not "cure" mental illness and hospitals gradually become warehouses, crammed with patients.
1905	Clifford Beers, Wall Street businessman, who is mentally ill and frequently hospitalized, founds the National Committee for Mental Hygiene, now the National Mental Health Association. He also authors A MIND THAT FOUND ITSELF.
1931	A building for the exclusive care of the criminally insane opened on grounds of Central State Hospital.
1940	NAZI Germany begins its euthanasia program to eliminate people with mental illness and retardation who are considered "life unworthy of life." Ultimately, in select asylums, 70,000 people are killed by starvation, injection, or gas.
1943	Tennessee's fourth state psychiatric hospital opens in Memphis.
1941-45	WWII focuses national concern on military losses from mental disorders. The U.S. Army learns that when "shell shocked" troops were treated quickly, they returned to combat sooner.
1946-1948	Community mental health clinics open in Chattanooga, Knoxville and Nashville, Tennessee.

1950	550,000 mentally ill people occupy psychiatric beds throughout the country; 7,400 in Tennessee.
1953	Tennessee Department of Mental Health, created by Governor Frank Clement, is one of the first such cabinet level departments in the nation.
	Discovery of DNA's double helix, the molecular structure that stores genetic information. This discovery and the development of computers eventually leads to the United States launching the Human Genome Project in 1990.
1954	Thorazine discovered to control symptoms of schizophrenia making it possible to care for many severely mentally ill people in the community. Schizophrenia is estimated to affect 1% of the general population.
1955	Mental Health Guidance Center of Middle Tennessee opens in Nashville. (In 1970, its name is changed to Dede Wallace Center).
1958	Tennessee Association of Mental Health Centers founded. (Name changed in 1995 to the Tennessee Association of Mental Health Organizations – TAMHO.) TAMHO is a trade association representing community service provider agencies.
1961	Moccasin Bend Psychiatric Hospital opens in Chattanooga, Tennessee.
1962	Re-Education Center (Cumberland House), for emotionally disturbed children opens in Nashville as a nationally recognized model program.
1963	Community Mental Health Centers Act signed into law by President John F. Kennedy establishes national goals and funding for constructing and staffing of community mental health centers across the United States. With this "bold new approach" deinstitutionalization becomes national policy.
	Division of Mental Retardation established in Tennessee Department of Mental Health (TDMH).
	Alcoholism programs transferred from Department of Public Health to TDMH.
1960-70s	The three rural centers, that in the late 1990's become part of Centerstone, open: • Harriet Cohn Mental Health Center – Clarksville, seven counties (1960). • Highland Rim Mental Health Center – Tullahoma, five counties (1967). • Columbia Area Mental Health Center – Columbia, eight counties (1964).
	Thirty-one community mental health centers eventually established in Tennessee.
	Deinstitutionalization is less than a success. Many mentally ill people are discharged from state hospitals without adequate community treatment and housing being available. Over time, homelessness and jail incarceration increase.
1975	TDMH renamed Tennessee Department of Mental Health and Mental Retardation (TDMHMR).
1979	National Alliance for the Mentally Ill founded in Wisconsin. (By 1998, 160,000 families are members).
1982	Community Initiative plan established by the TDMHMR to decrease state hospital beds and increase community funding and services.

1985	Tennessee Alliance for the Mentally Ill founded with membership composed mainly of families with people who have mental illness.
1988	Tennessee Mental Health Consumer's Association founded for members who are mental health consumers and others who support TMHCA's mission.
1990	The Human Genome Project begins with the goal of sequencing three billion letters of DNA. The search for genetic influences on mental illness accelerates.
1991	Alcohol and Drug Division of TDMHMR is transferred to the Tennessee Department of Health. The state plans to eventually put mental services into the Department of Health but this is prevented by the strong opposition of TAMHO and other advocacy groups.
1992	Tennessee's Master Plan is prepared to expand community services and funding and to further diminish use of hospitals. While the majority of people are now being successfully treated in the community, housing and psychological rehabilitation remain inadequate.
1994	TennCare established to manage care and control funding of Tennessee's Medicaid and uninsured population. This results in major changes in funding and leads to some community mental health centers forming legal affiliations. One center closes in 1997.
1996	The State "carves out" the management of mental health services from TennCare thus creating the TennCare Partner's Program. The State direct contracts with the Behavioral Health Organizations (BHOs) for the care and management of its former Medicaid behavioral health care population.
1997	February: Pinnacle Health, Inc. founded to manage Columbia Area Mental Health Center, Harriett Cohn Center, and Highland Rim Mental Health Center December: Pinnacle Health and Dede Wallace Center affiliate and establish Centerstone Community Mental Health Centers, Inc.
December 20, 1997	Nashville Banner reports people with mental illness are steadily increasing in the local jail. Growing concern in both Tennessee and nationally regarding the mentally ill filling the jails.
January, 1998	Average daily census at the five Tennessee state hospitals is down to 882. Private hospitals are increasingly used.
July, 1998	Luton Mental Health Services, founded in 1975, affiliates with Centerstone.
January, 2000	Centerstone begins management of the Elam Mental Health Clinic, founded in 1970, at Meharry Medical College.
June, 2000	Tennessee's mental health and mental retardation laws, Title 33, are totally revised. Department's name changed to Tennessee Department of Mental Health and Developmental Disabilities (TDMHDD). President Clinton announces completion of the rough draft of the human genome, "The Code of Life," increasing hope for an identification of genes that contribute to mental illness and for improved drugs and the ultimate potential of prevention.

July, 2000 Centerstone's five affiliates are fully merged.

January, 2001 Centerstone, the largest behavioral health provider in Tennessee, provides services for approximately 48,000 Tennesseans, residents in 26 counties in Middle Tennessee. These services are provided across 56 locations by approximately 1100 staff, and a $50 million budget. Research, telemedicine, integration with primary care are among many new commitments. The board establishes new mission and vision statements and selects "Everyone Matters" as Centerstone's motto.

The Future Some visions for Centerstone:

- Research becomes a major part of Centerstone, advancing knowledge, treatment and prevention.
- A Senior Services Division is established with specialized services for the elderly throughout the service area.
- Integration with primary care is so well developed that it provides a complete system of care.
- Centerstone's quality of care is consistently ranked high by national and state standards and by consumer and family satisfaction surveys.
- Telemedicine system is expanded throughout the service area linking psychiatric hospitals, emergency rooms and outpatient clinics.
- Centerstone is recognized for the involvement of consumers and family members in planning and delivery of mental health services.
- Centerstone's service area has one of the lowest rates of hospital utilization in the nation . A broad array of community services, emphasizing prevention and recovery, decreases the need for hospital treatment.
- In collaboration with other advocacy groups, Centerstone helps eliminate stigma about mental illness.

"I believe we will reach a point where we won't segregate our mentally ill and mentally retarded. We will recognize they are us."

-- Dr. Lloyd Elam
1978

George E. Spain
Revised March 6, 2002

1960's presentation
to mother's group

To become a mother you go through a great deal, and I think that it is because you go through so much that you become able to see with especial clearness certain fundamental principles of infant care, so that it takes years of study for those of us who are not mothers to get as far in understanding as you may get in the ordinary course of experience. You first get to know something of your baby's characteristics just through the movements he made in your womb. And during that time the baby got to know quite a lot about you through such experiences as meal time, your excitement, anger or happiness. Even in the womb your babies were each human beings unlike any other human beings and by the time they were born both you and they had shared numerous experiences, both unpleasant as well as pleasant. And all of this culminating at nine months in birth. No matter what occurs following this event the mother had experienced the heights of intimacy which no person could ever know with this human being. However, even you may need support at times because superstitions and old wives tales - some of them quite modern ones - come along and make you doubt your own feelings.

Even mothers have to learn how to be motherly by experience. I think it is much better if you look at it in that way. By experience mothers, as well as fathers, grow. If you look at it the other way and think you must work hard at books to learn how to be perfect mothers from the beginning, you will be on the wrong track. In the long run, what is needed are mothers as well as fathers who have found out how to believe in themselves. These mothers and their husbands build the best homes in which their children can grow and develop.

Since I know that for the most part all of the mothers here today have this faith in their own abilities it is not my course to tell you what to do in rearing your children and particularly in preparing them for school. Being a man, I can never really know what it is like to see wrapped up in a crib a bit of myself which has lived and moved within me, nor the other multitude of intimacies between a mother and child. Therefore, I cannot tell you exactly what to do in preparing your children for school or helping them with the numerous problems they encounter day by day. Rather I would like to attempt to explain what some of it means from the little peoples point of view. To prevent our giant stepping without even a may I into the world of a five to eight year old child we are duty bound to look at what has happened to him before this time. In this brief review of early development it is interesting to consider the child's emotional world from two powerful factors - love and hate, the latter including aggression, antagonism, hostility, anger, etc.

It has been generally agreed by those who study child development that the most important influence to the growth and maturing of a healthy personality in the child is sound relationship with both parents. His basic capacity for response and for forming and maintaining good emotional and social relationships throughout life is rooted and patterned in these early beginnings. His later reactions to the teachers and fellow students have for the most part been decided in his relationships at home. Hence the creative function of parents is by no means finished when the child is born. From the emotional point of view it has just begun. In much the same way the baby developed inside its mother, absorbing what was needed for physical maturing, so the mental life of the child feeds and grows upon the relationship with his parents. Our keynote for understanding the behavior of children is the acceptance of the long period of mental immaturity. Therefore to be successful as parents, fathers and mothers need the capacity to love their children for their potential and what is to come rather than feel affection for their lack of finish. We must always keep in mind that like ourselves each child is a different individual thereby developing differently. So that if one is a little slower in speech, toilet training, social response or any other area we do not attempt too vigorously to even up the inbalance. Much of the baby trails along in the toddler who frequently needs the privilege of being a baby. And so is true of the older child.

What is it like to be born and first experience life outside a world where everything is blissfully taken care of automatically? To be suddenly projected into a world where you are bombarded with noises, bright lights, smells and a smack on the bottom? Well maybe all of its so frightening and confusing that we don't remember it and maybe that is why we don't recall anythin that happens during our first few years. But even though we are unable to remember it is during the first year of life that the groundwork of our emotional development is laid. Babies, thank goodness, are born with some capacity to respond positively to another human being. After the first week of life they fix their gaze on the human face that approaches them with greater frequency than inanimate objects. At four to five weeks the look is often followed by a smile and gurgle. The hands of the child grope toward the feeder during the meal and by four or five months there is definite recognition of a familiar face. A basic relationship has been established. At this tender age it is not clearly love rather he needs his mother more to satisfy his hunger; she is a necessity for life. But the relationship between the infant and mother soon goes far beyond what is to be explained as necessary for the preservation of life. The child wants his mother near and longs for her even when hunger is satisfied and no dangers are threatening. We say the child loves his mother. The skill and tenderness with which feeding, bathing, dressing, holding and other activities are caried out contribute toward the child's first love feeling toward other persons who later can offer comfort and pleasure.

- 4 -

There finally comes, however, the moment when the child suddenly learns that his mother does not belong to him alone. He gradually realizes that others, the father and possibly brothers and sisters, also claim a right to her possession. Not only does he have to contend with this loss but also there is the beginning of the loss of freedom. Controls are placed on his greediness and his control of the world around him both of which revolved around his mouth. He eats like a little pig, bites, licks and tastes of everything, even people, and screams his demands when things aren't going well. Around age two when he has just begun gaining some control over those wobbly legs and arms and has a few words there comes the time when mother and father start pulling on the bridles. Training in cleanliness with the toilet being only one of the many demands which make him mad. His anger and aggressiveness is expressed through refusal to comply to parents demands, occasional tantrums, vigorous activity, and other means. He is very sensitive and parental understanding of this period and an occasional restrained participation in the child's rowdy activities adds greatly to the love feeling of the child for the parents. Self control over our own angry feelings when he refuses to comply is vitally necessary for the successful handling of aggressive activity. Our feelings are quickly picked up on and such reaction can easily result in alarm or additional anger. He is fascinated by the feelings within his own person and therefore his feelings, like his attention, are extremely distractable. However, if the relationship with the parents is a happy one and the training is a true education and not a rigid discipline, the successful establishment of cleanliness progresses easily.

Education of a child begins with the first day of life and with the completion of the second year he comes to realize that something is being demanded of him. Its universal aim is always to make out of the child a grown-up person who shall not be very different from the grown ups around him.

- 5 -

Before progressing to the third year I would like to re-emphasize what I mentioned in the beginning regarding development. Transition from one stage to the next is not sharply defined so that almost every child will progress or hold onto earlier reactions according to his own individual abilities. It is necessary to make allowances for incompleteness. The unorganized mind of the young infant is not ready to fit in the convenience of routine family life and his maturing may be endangered or supported by family activities. Parenthood is not an atonement but rather an enrichment. The complexity of the interactions between the mother and child and within the entire family cannot be reduced to rigid formulas. Love and understanding cannot be prescribed, and if they are not genuinely manifested, the most enlightened efforts to do what is best for the child may not be effective.

During these early years as the child improves his abilities and gains control over himself he gradually strives for independence. His curiosity in all things around him, his body and its functions is a first step toward his independence. His interest in his body during the third to fifth year is a part of every child's normal development. He is curious about functions of the body and asks questions which if ignored or for which he is punished can lead to a misunderstanding of himself and later on to feelings of guilt and shame about natural functions. Further strong disapproval of the child's most natural expression of bodily pleasure starts a rift in the relation with the parents and arouses a feeling of not being loved, which may have far reaching effects. Curiosity is a highly important stimulus to learning. Questions will be asked by every child whose parents do not have a forbidding attitude and when the replies are made without embarrassment but with frankness and do not go beyond the immediate question the child is satisfied. An element of deep trust is then added to the parent-child relationship.

During this same period the child usually develops a strong love for the parent of the opposite sex and an intense rivalry with the parent of the same sex. The boy becomes protective of the mother and wants much personal attention from her and at the same time is antagonistic to his father. The same is true of the little girl though her affection turns toward her father. This can be a very difficult period in the child's life and expert understanding and help is required of the parents. Success depends largely on their attitudes, on their deep love for each other and on the understanding they have shown through the early stages of the child's development.

Strange though it may seem aggression and anger are a necessary emotion in the life of human beings. It enables the child to gain his independence and reach maturity. It is necessary for the defense of his immature self, leting adults know when he is in pain or when he needs something to provide for his well being. It is highly important not to arouse and over stimualte these feelings. On the other hand the child who is left undirected with complete permissiveness is in actuality seriously unhappy due to the fears brought on by no restriction.

Finally we come to our five to eight year old and the enlarged world that kindergarten and school open up before them. My belaboring of the child's earlier feelings and drives was to enable us to see him at this point as the culmination of not only his own innate drives but the result of parental demands and expectations. The teacher does not have the enviable position of dealing with untilled ground. Each child brings with him a collection of characteristics, and reacts to the teacher in his own precise fashion. There is to be discovered in each child a perfectly definite constellation of hopes and fears, likes and dislikes, his own kind of jealousy and tenderness and his need for or rejection of love. The teacher is moving among already complex miniature personalities whom it is by no means easy to influence.

- 7 -

Do you remember the first day you began school? Mine is quite vivid as I was a week late due to some confusion of my parents on the day school opened. At that point in my life it was probably the most humiliating experience I had suffered. I was sure the teacher thought I was an idiot and the other children knew I was and of course as children will they let me know it.

There are two sides to the coin on a child's feelings about beginning school. In one way this is saying to the whole world "look at me, I'm really big now". You can see this in the cockiness of their walk, the way they sling their books or their all knowing expression. Of course this is also a mark for the other side for this is a second weaning and this time there is no mother or father around to help. For the first time he is all alone. Not only does he have to face the demands of the all powerful personnage of the teacher but also those of the children that surround him. His security depends somewhat on the skill with which he meets the two forces so essential to his sense of adequacy - his need to please the teacher, and his desire to be liked by the youngsters. All this while attempting new and challenging kinds of learning.

This is why he needed earlier successful and rewarding experiences at home particularly in his relationship with his parents. If he is secure in their love this new venture is not felt as a casting out into bondage. Rather he realizes in his own little way that this again is a step in helping him to become independent and eventually free himself into the adult world.

Burdened with the education received in the home the child is indeed anything but a blank sheet. The transformation that has taken place within him is amazing. Out of the creature so dependent upon others and to those around him almost intolerable, a more or less reasonable human being has been evolved. The school child who enters the classroom is therefore prepared to find that he is only one among many, and from this time on cannot count on any privileged position. He has learned something of social adaptation. Instead of continually seeking to gratify his desires, as formerly, he is now prepared to do what is required of him and to confine his pleasures to the times allowed for them. His interests and curiosity if not impaired when initially expressed are now transformed into a thirst for knowledge and a love for learning. In pleace of the revelations and explanations which he longed for earlier he is now prepared to obtain a knowledge of letters and numbers.

The fifth through approximately tenth years are quiet ones relatively speaking, and therefore good for the beginning of formalized education. The instinctual impulses slow down permitting the child to begin training his intellect. The child begins to see his parents in a more reasonable light and while his feeling of love for them is maintained he continues his striving for freedom.

The nature of the child's relationship to his parents is often revealed for the first time during this period. If a child has learned through day by day homelife that adults are accepting, friendly persons, even if at times they impose restrictions, he will turn to new contacts with other adults with the confidence created by these early experiences. This confidence may at first be overshadowed by the timidity that is the natural part of an unfamilar experience.

Some of the love originally felt for the parents is transfered onto the teacher giving the child a desire to do good work and behave properly which he realizes will please her. Also it is not infrequent that some of the anger or hostility felt for the parents is carried over to the teacher. A wise teacher, however, like a wise parent has some understanding of such behavior and makes allowances. Again this does not mean that aggression should go unchecked rather limitations should be geared to the individual child's capacity to accept it without being overwhelmed.

Most children by this time are able to tolerate this separation from their parents without great difficulty, however, some regression such as thumb sucking, soiling or occasional irritability should not be taken as severe disturbance. After all the child is under a strain and should not be expected to handle this feat without some expression of his resentment toward his new world.

Severe difficulties in learning, if the child has average intellectual capacity, are usually the result of disturbances experienced in preceeding levels of development. Repression of curiosity in earlier years often results in repression of the desire to learn. Learning which is normally a pleasure then becomes a forbidden pleasure. The small child, eager to learn, does so with an enthusiasm and zest that can be associated only with an aggressive striving toward gaining a goal. Children who have come to fear their aggressions will then fear the aggressiveness inherent in learning.

The first three years of school for a child can and should fulfill the promise that he will "feel big". First grade is a major step into that outside world in which every youngster must eventually live with increasing independence and self sufficiency. By the age of 8 or 9 children have usually achieved the smooth competence and self assurance that mark them as fully established in the middle years of childhood. The successful overcoming of hurdles that mark this time of growth will only lead to further growth. He feels big and looks forward to more school hurdles with the air of the conquering hero.

In Vanity Fair William Thackeray declares that "mother is the name for God in the lips and hearts of little children". Simply through being devoted to your children you with your husbands support make an immense contribution to society. If the magnitude of your contribution is accepted, it follows that every man or woman who is sane, every man or woman who feels to be a person in the world and for whom the world means something, every happy person, is in infinite debt to a woman. At a time when as an infant we all knew nothing about dependence, there was absolute dependence upon our mothers.

December 11, 1968

Dr. Joseph Weinreb
Department of Psychiatry
Vanderbilt University Hospital
21st Avenue South
Nashville, Tennessee

Dear Dr. Weinreb:

At your request the enclosed proposals of Committee II on the Conference On Child Care is presented for enclusion in the total report. None of the members of this committee were participants in developing the original proposals at the first conference.

If there are any questions regarding this report please contact me or Mrs. Erline Gore who served on the committee and who read the proposals to the conference.

I would personally like to express the appreciation of the Maury County Mental Health Clinic for the invitation to the conference. We particularly appreciated your kindness to Judge John Stanton.

Sincerely,

George Spain

George Spain
Psychiatric Social Worker

GS/bwl

Enc: 2

MAURY COUNTY
Mental Health Clinic
Memorial Building
West Seventh Street
Telephone 388-6653
COLUMBIA, TENNESSEE
38401

Conference On Child Care

December 5-6, 1968

The committee that met to review Section II suggests the following revisions and additions. See, for comparision the original statement proposed by the initial conference committee.

2. Services for the physically, intellectually and emotionally handicapped should include:

A. Remedial medical measures.
B. Consider the establishment of regional child development centers for comprehensive evaluations of all types of handicapped children. (Such as University of Tennessee Medical Center, Memphis; Vanderbilt University Hospital, Nashville)
C. Development of services for the preschool handicapped child. (Improved evaluation services, in such programs as headstart, referrals and treatment if necessary)
D. Additional educative and supportive services for parents of handicapped children. There is a need for increasing and improving services that are actually provided for the patient and family within the home.
E. Improved and expanded educational programs for handicappped children that realistically prepare him for employment needs in our present society.
    1. Prevocational training programs for primary grade children such as are in operation within the Memphis area which combines both vocational rehabilitation and education services.
F. Improved vocational training programs that realistically prepare handicapped children for employment needs.
G. Develop adequate foster care programs which are presently non-existant for handicapped children.
H. A system of hospital and boarding school facilities to meet the variety of needs of children who cannot be cared for at home.
    1. Adequate medical care to prevent or minimize later crippling.
    2. Psychiatric treatment services for all children where

FOR THE EMOTIONAL AND SOCIAL PROBLEMS OF EVERYDAY LIVING

emotional state requires it. Including: inpatient, outpatient, day care, night care and halfway house programs.

3. Special residential schools for emotional disturbed children that includes day, night and interim care.
4. Hospital facilities for all retarded who need such care.
5. Other special training facilities for the educable and trainable retarded of all ages.
6. Out-patient department facilities for all the above when this service will suffice or as a later follow up.

The committee also suggests the following services that could benefit all children and families in Tennessee.

A. The State should compile and maintain comprehensive directories of services available for children including both public and private. Each State department that provides services for children might provide a directory relevant to its own programs.

B. Utilization of communication media for increased education of the public as to the overall needs of children. If energetically pursued local television stations might provide free public service time such as arranged recently for education on cigarettee smoking. However, the orininality provided by professional advertising agencies should be considered to present the information with greatest impact and relevance.

C. Improved recruitment programs for professional and para professional personnel. This should be given immediate attention due to the present interest of Americans youth for improved racial conditions in this country. However, in the past, this has been done in a rather irratic disorganized manner in Tennessee so that the State might be considered as the agency to develop a more comprehensive coverage.

George Spain

George Spain, Chairman

GS/bwl

Presentation to the Finance, Ways & Means Committee of the Tennessee General Assembly.

January 30, 1996

~~Subject~~ Tennessee's: Community M H Centers.

¶ I am a native Tennesseean. What I say is ~~meant~~ not only for this committee but also for all our other legislators, the Administration ~~Governor, the dept. of~~ M.H. and the people of Tennessee.

~~One of~~ Last year I heard m.h. presentations made to this committee which for the most part gave broad statistics + detailed columns on money. I want to present something about real people + something about one mental health center, what it does + who does it. then, I hope, you will better understand why the State, along with local government, + the people we serve must, together, increase their support of the community mental health centers.

One of my earliest memories, when I was between 4-6 yrs, was a visit to the old Davidson County Asylum to visit an aunt. All I remember were the bars and a man walking down the hall who looked like a guard. Right or wrong the memory is not of a hospital but of a prison.

Years later, as a student, I trained there and ~~summer~~ saw patients spending most, if not all, of their days sitting in wards that still vaguely resembled a prison. + I saw a female patient choked unconscious with towels + then helped carry her to a ~~[illegible]~~ lock up room.

The next year I worked in the summer in the Cooper building at Central State. There to care for several hundred patients was one M.D. who was not a psychiatrist, one nurse + a hand full of aides. My job was to try to find families of men + women who had had no mail, no visits for 5, 10, 20 years. One man, slightly retarded, in no way violent had been there over 10 yrs + every summer his family would take him home, near Memphis to pick cotten + after that bring him back. Many patients recieved electric shock treatment. Once ~~One day~~ when there were no aides to help, another student + myself helped hold patients arms + legs while ~~the~~ shock treatment was given.

For the most part we have come a long way since then. State Hospital care + treatment is more humane + better + available to more patients + the overall standard has improved. I support the States continuing effort to improve State Hospital treatment ~~the care~~ + recognize accreditation is a must for these Hospitals. I recognize that the Community M.H. Centers are not able to handle or treat all patients in their In Patient Units + therefore the State Hospitals are necessary to care for those few patients that are extremely aggressive or who require many months of treatment.

~~However~~, the steady improvement of care in State Hospitals is directly related to the development of Tennessee's Community M H + their assumption of ~~treatment~~ of patients who would have gone to the Hospital Centers. In 1968 the average daily population at Central State was 3788. On December 5, 1975 there were 1205 patients - A third less.

~~During the years from~~ Since 1968 to present there has been an appreciable growth in the Community M.H. Centers throughout Tennessee

-4

The Columbia Area MH Center began as the Maury Co MH Clinic in 1964. In July 1972 with receipt of Federal funds it expanded services to 8 counties with a total of 150,000 people. There are now out pt. clinics in each of the 8 counties + a 10 bed in pt. unit in Maury Co. Hospital + 24 hour emergency service located in Columbia

What has this Center with the help of the Community accomplished? In 1968 there were XX 244 of our people ~~were~~ admitted to Central State. ~~+~~ 262 were traveling long distances from their homes to Central State for OP. follow up. A total of 506 were being cared for at Central State In 1974 only 86 people (⅓) were admitted there from our area - a 65% cut in admissions, + none were going for out pt. care. We admitted to our unit 125 people whose average length of stay was 9 days. ~~and~~ We are now following over 400 people - most of whom previously would have returned to the CSH OP Clinic

In the last 3 yrs 32 elderly patients have XX been transferred from Central State to Nursing Homes in Maury County ~~+~~ where we ~~have~~ see them regularly

-5

their families have been located + most now receive regular visits. Our doctor + nurse see them ~~regularly~~ monthly + the nurse takes them out more frequently for rides + picnics. Even with varying degrees of senility they are less withdrawn + more responsive to the world around them. Their physical care is markedly improved.

We assisted the magistrates in closing the M.C. Poor Farm + in transfering these people + several of whom had been to Central State + to Nursing Homes + continue to provide follow up care to several of them

In 1975 we saw approximately 1400 new people for mental health services + had ~~around 2500~~ over 2000 total people recieving services. We work in 4 county school systems providing evaluations of children + consultation to teachers + parents. Competency + child abuse evaluations are provided along with consultation to Juvenile Judges. We spend much time in jails + at the Turney Center for Youthful Offender in ~~Only, Tennessee~~ Hickman County where we provide all their required psychiatric evaluations + some direct ~~treatment~~.

Through the 8 county m.h. clinics we are the major agency providing marital + family counseling. Many of our clients have alcohol problems + may be detoxified at the hospital or treated at the local clinics. During the past year 100 people have gone through our DUI school at CSCC. —6

These accomplishments have been made with major support from the community - both financial + with time + help from many people. The ~~actual operation~~ actual services are now being provided with only 22 professionals. Because of diminishing funds from the Federal + State government by this summer we will have cut 4 ~~2 other~~ positions which were unfilled + 2 which were filled. ~~I believe~~ We have reached our limit in cuts if we are to continue what ~~we are doing~~ to properly serve the people in our area. 22 professional + 18 admin + cler people are very few ~~stretched thin in covering 8 counties + 150,000 people~~ to operate 8 clinics, an in pt unit, 24 hr emergency service, partial hospitalization + to provide consultation + education for 150,000 people

Our county + city officials have given steady increases in the past but are beginning to express hesitancy in how much more they can give. Our Federal grant (now $148,000)

-7

ends June, 1980. Our income from client fees & insurance has doubled in 2 yrs. because of more increased expectations for them to assume ~~some~~ responsibility. ~~However~~ Because most of our clients are poor or low income & even ~~with~~ with some increase from local government ~~these~~ we will not be able to maintain our present level ~~a good record~~ of service within coming years without the State assuming some part of the cost.

What I have said about the Columbia Center applies to the other MH Centers. ~~In total, last~~ This year, we were cut a total of $800,000 & A recent survey of the Centers showed a need for $725,627 from the State for 1976-77 just to maintain present service.

The progressive history of MH in Tennessee I have seen & ~~been~~ having had a part ~~of~~ in it I know we have been moving in the right direction. In a very few years each county should have its own m.h. clinic & inpt services should be expanded in areas where they are non-existant. ~~By 1980~~ We should continue to steadily ~~to~~ cut the State Hospital populations so that better treatment can be provided their patients ~~at least to a third of their present levels~~. Retardation Centers are major need particularly in rural areas

The Community m h centers are accomplishing the original reasons for their existance. While recognizing they must operate c greater financial efficiently + ~~business~~ there comes a time, + it is now, that increasing cuts not only impair the operation of the Centers but eventually lead to a slide back to our past history.

George Spain, ACSW
Executive Director
CAMHC

1980

Here it begins ☆

INTRODUCTION

Chains and lock-up rooms in family homes, living in caves, jails, and poor houses were the conditions of many mentally ill Tennesseans during the first thirty-six years of our state. Faced with the terrible conditions of these unfortunate people the state legislature on October 19, 1832 first assumed responsibility for helping the mentally ill. Ten thousand dollars was appropriated so that a suitable hospital could be erected in this state for their comfort and security. Since the opening of this first hospital in 1840 state government has maintained a major responsibility for the caring of the mentally ill. By the early 1960's things had changed from what was originally intended, as the five-state hospitals had become overcrowded warehouses where on the average day 7,500 Tennesseans were kept with fewer legal rights than most prisoners. This insidious trend began to reverse in 1964 because of new medicines, legal changes, education, advocacy by Mental Health Association members, general societal changes, and treatment provided in communities by private practioners and the community mental health programs. In the 1940's outpatient mental health clinics were established in our four largest cities. These have now increased to 33 mental health centers which are responsible for the operations of clinics in most of our 95 counties along with many other services to help the severely mentally ill and emotionally troubled along with those having problems with alcohol and drugs. Now most Tennesseans who need mental health services can be helped in their home county or nearby. From the 2,100 people served in 1955 by the first four clinics there are now 100,000 helped each year by community mental health centers. This has enabled the closure of all the outpatient clinics once operated by the state hospitals. Since 1964 the daily number of patients in these hospitals has steadily declined largely due to the centers acceptance of responsibility for helping thousands return to the community and the prevention of admissions through the use of local programs. The overall result is that care and treatment is better and more humane while family and work ties are less disrupted. Now on an average day there are only 2,300 people in the five hospitals. Within the next few years we should expect to do much more with the ultimate result that state hospitals become a part of our history. We should also expect a major change in state funding of which almost 80% goes to the state hospitals while the majority of severely mentally ill now live in the community. Control of non-profit community mental health centers by local boards of directors rather than by the state has resulted in services being more directly related to community needs. It has produced a check and balance system of accountability on centers which is generally not found in state or private directed services. Local control has resulted in thousands of Tennesseans volunteering their time as board members. These people have increasingly influenced positive changes in community attitudes about mental illness. They along with Mental Health Association volunteers have provided leadership in obtaining the local support needed for severely mentally ill people to return and remain in their communities. The boards have played the major role in the centers obtaining local government funding and are increasingly using their influence to obtain private donations and grants. The circle of responsibility for helping the mentally ill has almost completed its full circle from community to state hospital and now back to the community. As always this health and social change is influenced by and reflected in the economy and political mood of the nation. Across the nation state appropriations have essentially remained with state hospitals even though most of the severely mentally ill now live in the community. In some states the care and treatment of these people appear to be going backwards. Though this is not yet true in Tennessee, it could occur if state funds are steadily shifted away to the general fund with the majority of what remains going to state hospitals. While in recent years the legislature's intent has been to appreciably increase funding to community programs successful in decreasing the number of patients in state hospitals, yet the fact is that the shift of funds is not keeping up with the shift of patients. Without basic reform this major problem will probably continue. Answers to questions such as the following will indicate whether the mental health system in Tennessee continues essentially unchanged or whether planned basic reform will be set into motion.

1. Is major reform in Tennessee's mental health system necessary in order to make major improvements in care and treatment?

2. Should the state continue to provide direct services?

Could these services be improved using existing funds by changes in administrative control of state hospitals and by shifting more hospital services to the community?

3. Are Tennessee community mental health centers willing to accept greater legal and service responsibilities for the mental health needs of the people in their areas?

4. Is the state willing to continue to support local control of community mental health centers and at the same time provide state funds on the front end so that the centers may either purchase needed services from Mental Health Institutes or develop them locally?

5. How can representatives of all mental health care contribute to the discussion and debate needed to develop mutually shared goals for a comprehensive state-wide plan that strengthens a working relationship between private and non-

profit providers which improves services?

6. How can existing state service funds and unused state mental health institute buildings and lands be saved for more equal geographic distribution to community services?

7. Is the Tennessee Association of Mental Health Centers willing to accept the leadership responsibility for developing a detailed plan which will bring about major improvements in mental health services?

DEVELOPMENT AND PHILOSOPHY OF THE PLAN

In an effort to address these questions the long-range planning committee of the Tennessee Association of Mental Health Centers was appointed. This committee has been meeting for a couple of years discussing questions relative to the future of mental health in Tennessee. As a result of these discussions we felt that a planning document needed to be drafted that outlined a specific course of action for our association over the next several years. We were searching for a plan that would help the mental health system in Tennessee in several ways. First, we were interested in a plan that would help maximize the limited amount of resources that are going to be available in the coming years for mental health services. We wanted a commitment for the development of the most humane and least restricted treatments to be a major goal. Third, we felt that our plan should be consistent with the national as well as the Tennessee mood which has shifted toward an emphasis on local control of governmental and human service functions. Fourth, we wanted a plan that would be cost competitive with other mental health providers. Fifth, we wanted a plan that had assurances for accountability and quality control to insure that the best possible mental health care would be provided to the people in Tennessee. Last, we wanted a system that promoted compatibility between the private and non-profit mental health centers and the general health care system in Tennessee. These goals could be summarized as follows:

a) maximize mental health resources;

b) insure humane least restricted treatment;

c) be consistent with the national mood toward decentralization:

d) enable the private, non-profit mental health centers to be cost competitive;

e) to promote volunteerism;

f) to enhance accountability, quality control, and quality mental health treatment.

To accomplish these goals will require a major redefinition and overhaul of the mental health system in Tennessee. The central concept guiding this restructuring and the main theme of this planning document is that the major responsibility for mental health care is now at the local community level. This responsibility has been assumed gradually over time with the deinstitutionalization program implemented by the Tennessee Department of Mental Health. This transfer of responsibility (and patients) has occurred without sufficient state resources being reallocated from the state-run institutional programs to sufficiently provide the needed community support programs.

OBJECTIVES/ACTIONS

1. TAMHC will approve a long range planning document for implementation according to a specified time frame.
2. The TAMHC in concert with TDMH will prepare a revision of the mental health statutes to be consistent with the assumptions stated on pages 11 and 12.
3. Adopt a position on equalization of funding for geographic populations.
4. The conduit for state legislative appropriations for all direct mental health services in Tennessee will be community mental health centers.
5. Mental Health Center directors and the Regional Mental Health Institute superintendent, along with their respective boards, will develop a plan with TDMH for the administration and utilization of the regional mental health institute.
6. The role of TDMHwill be defined as the primary monitoring entity for mental health services on behalf of the legislature and state administration.
7. A study will be conducted of institute facilities and lands. Unused properties will be leased or sold with the revenue redistributed to communities for housing and vocational improvements for the severely mentally ill.
8. TAMHC in consultation with TDMH will develop a plan for restructuring center service areas and/or administrative structures, that considers population, geography, political boundaries, and improvement in community services.
9. A plan of objectives will be established for funding and implementation of research pertinent to the delivery of community based mental health services.
10. A plan will be developed for soliciting the support and cooperation of other non-profit and private mental health service providers.
11. In cooperation with the Tennessee Mental Health Association a plan will be developed to educate the public about community based care and services, the mental health needs of the state and to further reduce the stigma associated with mental illness.
12. The TAMHC Executive Committee will develop a plan and committee for organizing the TAMHC for the accomplishment of these objectives.
13. A TAMHC committee will develop successful, example models which will fulfill the mental health needs of a given geographic area and on an ongoing basis assure quality care.
14. A plan will be developed for the training, hiring, and relocation of qualified state employees to work in community mental health programs.

George Spain
1980

HOUSE JOINT RESOLUTION NO. 400

By Bragg

A RESOLUTION to direct the Department of Mental Health and Mental Retardation to study needs for funding of community mental health centers and mental retardation programs and to report its findings and recommendations to the Governor, the Speaker of the House of Representatives, the Speaker of the Senate, and the Board of Trustees of the Department of Mental Health and Mental Retardation.

WHEREAS, the State of Tennessee has responsibility to plan for the needs and care of its citizens who may be mentally ill, mentally retarded, or developmentally disabled, and

WHEREAS, the General Assembly created the Department of Mental Health and Mental Retardation for the better treatment, training, and welfare of the mentally ill, the mentally retarded, and the developmentally disabled in this state, and

WHEREAS, the General Assembly recognizes that optimal treatment and habilitation of the mentally ill, the mentally retarded, and the developmentally disabled can best be accomplished in the home community rather than in large, centralized institutions, and

WHEREAS, there are now more than 130 community mental health centers and community mental retardation programs for the mentally ill, the mentally retarded, and the developmentally disabled in Tennessee, and

WHEREAS, these facilities and programs play an integral role in providing mental health and mental retardation care to citizens of this state, and

WHEREAS, it is widely recognized that the cost of providing services and care to the mentally ill, the mentally retarded, and the developmentally disabled has increased because of rising costs due to inflation and increasing demands for services and care, and

Resolutions] PUBLIC ACTS, 1976 1741

WHEREAS, state funding of community mental health centers and community mental retardation programs has not increased, and

WHEREAS, there appear to be inequities in the distribution of state appropriations to community mental health centers and community mental retardation programs across the state; now, therefore,

BE IT RESOLVED BY THE HOUSE OF REPRESENTATIVES OF THE EIGHTY-NINTH GENERAL ASSEMBLY OF THE STATE OF TENNESSEE, THE SENATE CONCURRING, That the department of mental health and mental retardation be directed to study the needs and determine the method for distribution of funds to community mental health centers and community mental retardation programs in Tennessee so that per capita equity and local effort may be established.

BE IT FURTHER RESOLVED, That the department within the course of its study shall: clearly identify the service areas within the state; identify the total number of persons served within each service area; identify the total number of persons served within each individual community mental health center; identify the total number of persons per center classified as mentally ill, mentally retarded and developmentally disabled; identify local governments cost maintenance levels for each community mental health and mental retardation center.

BE IT FURTHER RESOLVED, That the department of mental health and mental retardation report its findings and recommendations to the Governor of the State of Tennessee, to the Speaker of the House of Representatives, to the Speaker of the Senate and to the Board of Trustees of the Department of Mental Health and Mental Retardation, by October 1, 1976.

1742 **PUBLIC ACTS, 1976** [Resolutions

ADOPTED: March 16, 1976

Ned R. McWherter,
SPEAKER OF THE HOUSE OF REPRESENTATIVES

John S. Wilder,
SPEAKER OF THE SENATE

APPROVED: March 29, 1976

Ray Blanton,
GOVERNOR

(615) 388-6653

COLUMBIA AREA MENTAL HEALTH CENTER
OF CENTRAL TENNESSEE

TROTWOOD AVENUE
P. O. BOX 1119
COLUMBIA, TENNESSEE 38401

March 30, 1981

Mr. Ed Holton, Chief of Police
Columbia Police Department
707 N. Main Street
Columbia, Tennessee 38401

Dear Chief Holton:

I am formally registering a complaint against Officer Maurice Parham because of his rude and unprofessional behavior to a Center professional, Mrs. Nancy Pigg and me on March 26, 1981.

The events which led up to the matter began earlier in the day when Mrs. [redacted] attempted to cash large checks at two branch banks of Middle Tennessee Bank. Having only a very limited amount in her account, she was refused. In the afternoon she attempted to have two large checks cashed at the main office, was refused, and referred to Mr. Jimmy Couch. She informed Mr. Couch that Mrs. Betty Ford and some other well known person had deposited funds in her account and were waiting for her at the Nashville airport. When Mr. Couch said this was not so and therefore they could not cash the checks, she said, "well if you won't help me I have an atom bomb in the car and am going to blow the bank up". She left and a relative, Mr. [redacted] came to Mr. Couch and explained that he needed to get her to the Mental Health Center but was afraid she would jump out of the car. He also related that once in the past she had a shotgun and was going to shoot her husband while he was in bed but had the wrong gauge shell. Mr. Couch called Mrs. Pigg, relayed the above information, and requested our help.

At 2:00 P.M. Mrs. Pigg and I drove past the Bank and saw Mrs. [redacted] standing by her car. We came to the Police Department and requested assistance in picking her up in order to bring her to the Mental Health Center. We explained we would initially approach Mrs. [redacted] and attempt to get her to go voluntarily but we needed police assistance because of her threats and the possibility of her physically attacking us. Mr. [redacted] had come in to the Department and said he did not know if she had a weapon in her purse but that it was possible. Thinking that a warrent was needed, Sergeant Coleman and Assistant Chief Troop wanted clarification on this before proceeding. While we believed the warrant was not required according to Tennessee Code Anno. 33-603 (see enclosure), Mrs. Pigg agreed to call Judge William Fraser to clarify the matter.

While waiting for Judge Fraser to return the call, Mrs. Pigg and I were in the front room where Officer Parham was standing. He had heard much of what was going on. I asked him would he help me if Mrs. [redacted] attacked me?. With no emotion he

FOR THE EMOTIONAL AND SOCIAL PROBLEMS OF EVERYDAY LIVING

said, "I won't lay a hand on her". I said, "you mean if she attacks me you won't help?" He said, "No." I repeated my question and again in an "I could care less tone"said "No" and turned and walked out. As he was leaving I angrily made some comments about his rudeness and unprofessionalism.

Almost immediately the call from Judge Fraser came saying Mrs. [redacted] could be picked up without a warrant. Mrs. Pigg and I, at our request, first approached Mrs. [redacted] with Assistant Chief Troop and Sergeant Coleman approaching from the other side. After a few confused responses by Mrs. [redacted], she attempted to slam the door on us and we took hold of her arms and were immediately assisted by the two officers. Assistant Chief Troop and I took her to the car driven by Officer Parham who,followed by Mrs. Pigg and I and Sergeant Coleman, went to the Mental Health Center.

In a matter of minutes, Dr. Robert Reed talked with Mrs. [redacted] at the patrol car and signed emergency commitment papers. The ambulance service was contacted to provide transportation to Middle Tennessee Mental Health Institute.

While waiting for the ambulance, I went over to Officer Parham and told him that I wanted to apologize for blowing up and getting angry but his rudeness and unwillingness to help made me angry. He said nothing. Twice more he refused to respond and again I blew my stack, shook a fountain pen in his face and told him I was going to register a complaint against him.

Now in comparison, let me compliment Assistant Chief Troop and Sergeant Coleman. Even though they were concerned about needing a warrant, they were gentlemen, professional, and indicated a willingness to help as soon as they were sure about the warrant. This has always been my experience with these men who reflect well on your Department and their profession. I compliment them just as greatly as I condenm Officer Parham.

I personally cannot tolerate rudeness and disrespect from anyone, but especially from another "professional" and will not tolerate it from or to our staff at the Center. As our two staffs are frequently in contact and occasionally there are misunderstandings regarding the law in dealing with mentally ill people, we simply must maintain mutual respect and a willingness to help each other. I have a high regard for the Columbia Police and Sheriff's Departments. I would not push this matter if I did not consider it serious and wonder how Officer Parham might treat others in the community. Both Mrs. Pigg and I will be glad to meet with you to discuss this further if you wish. I, at least, hope we will receive a letter of apology from Officer Parham.

Sincerely,

George Spain

George Spain, MSW
Executive Director

GS:df

Enclosure

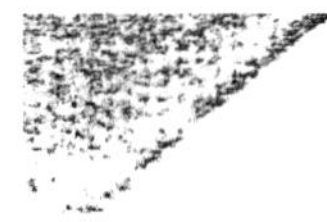

spouse, parent or legal guardian, or a licensed physician may file the request with the consent of the patient.

Within forty-eight (48) hours after receipt of the request, unless a petition for judicial hospitalization of the patient has been filed, the superintendent shall release the patient. If, however, the forty-eight (48) hour period expires on a Saturday, Sunday or legal holiday, the superintendent shall release the patient not later than noon of the next succeeding day which is not a Saturday, Sunday or legal holiday.

The superintendent may release any patient hospitalized under this section whenever he determines that the patient has recovered or that his continued hospitalization is no longer advisable or beneficial. [Acts 1965, ch. 38, § 37; 1974 (Adj. S.), ch. 802, § 43; 1975, ch. 248, § 14; 1976 (Adj. S.), ch. 763, § 5.]

33-602. [Repealed.]

33-603. Persons posing a likelihood of serious harm—Custody and hospitalization procedures.—(a) Any state, county or municipal officer authorized to make arrests in Tennessee or any licensed physician or licensed psychologist, when all reasonable efforts have been made to contact a licensed physician in the county and no such physician is available to conduct the examination within eight (8) hours of the first effort to contact a licensed physician, who has reason to believe that an individual is mentally ill and, because of this illness, poses a likelihood of serious harm if he is not immediately detained may, without a warrant, take such individual into custody. The phrase "likelihood of serious harm," for this section means (1) a substantial risk of physical harm to the person himself as manifested by evidence of threats of, or attempt at, suicide or serious bodily harm; or (2) a substantial risk of physical harm to other persons as manifested by evidence of homicidal or other violent behavior or evidence that others are placed in reasonable fear of violent behavior and serious physical harm to them.

If the individual is taken into custody by anyone other than a licensed physician or licensed psychologist, when all reasonable efforts have been made to contact a licensed physician in the county and no such physician is available to conduct the examination within eight (8) hours of the first effort to contact a licensed physician, he shall be taken immediately to the nearest available licensed physician or licensed phychologist, when all reasonable efforts have been made to contact a licensed physician in the county and

BILL RICHARDSON
REPRESENTATIVE

MAURY COUNTY
64TH DISTRICT

403 OAKWOOD DRIVE
COLUMBIA, TENNESSEE 38401
(615) 388-7753

38 LEGISLATIVE PLAZA
NASHVILLE, TENNESSEE 37219
(615) 741-3993

House of Representatives
State of Tennessee

NASHVILLE

SECRETARY
GOVERNMENT OPERATIONS

MEMBER OF COMMITTEES
TRANSPORTATION
CALENDAR AND RULES

March 17, 1982

Mr. George Spain
Columbia Area Mental Health Center
of Central Tennessee
Trotwood Avenue
Post Office Box 1119
Columbia, Tennessee 38401

Dear George:

The Government Operations Committees of the House and Senate have reviewed the Department of Mental Health. We have expressed concern over the cost of maintaining and operating the mental health institutes in light of a steadily declining population. We believe the Regional concept is working and has worked to such an extent that it is possible to consider a phase out or consolidation of some institutes. With that in mind, we have prepared a request(enclosed) that the Department supply the committees with certain information in order that we might make a sound judgment.

You have collected many facts and figures over the years and are the most knowledgable person I know in this area.

Please reveiw our proposal and make any comments. We are not going to limit our study. We do intend to move with caution in our evaluation as the political pressure can be great if any institution is singled out. We want any decisions to be on a practical rather than a political basis.

Sincerely,

Bill Richardson

BILL RICHARDSON

enc -1-

(615) 388-6653

COLUMBIA AREA MENTAL HEALTH CENTER
OF CENTRAL TENNESSEE

TROTWOOD AVENUE
P. O. BOX 1197
COLUMBIA, TENNESSEE 38401

February 19, 1982

Mr. Benjamin Dishman, Assistant Commissioner
Administrative Services
Tenn. Dept. of Mental Health & Mental Retardation
James K. Polk Office Building
505 Deaderick Street
Nashville, Tennessee 37219

Dear Ben:

Thank you for the explanation on the proposed reduction and your interest in possible long range goals for a major restructuring of the state's mental health system.

While I was glad to learn that the potential reduction is considerably less than I originally understood, I remain opposed to any cut since we have not only fulfilled our obligation according to the contract but have continued to reduce our area's use of the Institute.

Since we receive no special indigency hospitalization funding we are absorbing this major increasing cost as part of our total budget. As we have arranged for more and more patients from this and other areas to be discharged to our care in the community and as we put more manpower, time and money into preventing their regression and readmission to the Institute, the strain on us is at times almost overwhelming. What we are doing is working but to keep it up we simply must have more staff and money. Local government has just about reached its limit (about $1.00 per capita) and we squeeze and squeeze patient fees and third party sources but this will allow for only minimal growth. I see our staff working the hardest it has in my 13 years here and as we already priortize the severely mentally ill, what are we to do different and where are we to turn for the major infusion of money we need to care for more discharged patients?

It has been my belief, based on our experience here, that:

1. Centers with proper planning, commitment, and funding on the front end of all State appropriations (at present levels), on a per capita basis, can assume total responsibility for the mental health needs in their area.

2. The State can get out of direct service and have the Institutes run privately but reduced to much smaller sizes than at present - serving only

FOR THE EMOTIONAL AND SOCIAL PROBLEMS OF EVERYDAY LIVING

a very limited area. For example, MTMHI might need only one building to serve Davidson County. Centers would pay the Institutes if they used them otherwise all the money would go to community services.

3. The Department would provide overall assistance in planning and would be mainly the regulatory agency for State government.

I know some of the problems faced in such total change but if we all, the Department and Centers, worked together on it I believe it could be achieved in time. Most important in all of this is that it would be a far better way to treat not only the severely mentally ill but it would also improve services for everyone, whether psychotic, neurotic, or having problems with alcohol or drugs or just in adjusting to life.

As a member of the Association of Centers' Long Range Planning Committee I would like to have your response to these ideas. If you believe they are not just pipe dreams but are worthy of accomplishing, I would like to hear your suggestions and ideas as we are soon to begin meeting on specific plans. If you have not already done so, let me suggest that you read The Death of the Asylum by John A. Talbot, published by Grune and Stratton in 1978. Based on history, national studies and the author's own experience his conclusions should be considered by those in State Government and Community Mental Health as they plan for the future.

It is my belief that the Department and Centers waste entirely too much energy and brain power in attacking and defending gnats when if we worked together we might make one of those rare historical strides forward in caring for the mentally ill.

Sincerely,

George

George Spain, MSW
Executive Director

GS:df

Enclosures

cc: David Moore
Doug Varney
Don Finch

(615) 388-6653

COLUMBIA AREA MENTAL HEALTH CENTER
OF CENTRAL TENNESSEE

TROTWOOD AVENUE
P. O. BOX 1197
COLUMBIA, TENNESSEE 38401

December 28, 1982

Representative J. B. Napier
1119 Trotwood Avenue
Columbia, Tennessee 38401

Dear J. B. :

Knowing you are probably being contacted by many people with special concerns which the Legislature may soon focus upon, I want to put in a word for the severely mentally ill. I appreciate what you have already done in giving of your time to help our Center. Now as a state legislator your voice and vote will influence the state's future commitment to helping those who have major handicaps in making it in life because of their mental illness.

During the past 20 years a historical change, due to the development of new medicines and community mental health centers, has shifted the emphasis of care and treatment from our five state hospitals to community centers. For example, in 1962 our center's eight county area had over 420 people a day in state hospitals and in 1982 we were down to 40, a 90% decrease. The enclosed graph shows this decrease as it relates to the development of services in the area.

Statewide the decrease for the total patient population for the state hospitals has gone from 7,500 a day to less than 2,000. At today's costs for hospitalization Tennessee would likely be bankrupt if it was still responsible for 7,500 patients a day.

The problem which we need your help on is to influence the Legislature and Administration to shift more state funds from the Mental Health Institutes (hospitals) to where most of the patients now are - the community. Year after year the majority of mental health savings have either been diverted to the general fund or remained in the Institute budgets. More of these funds must come to community mental health centers to increase and improve services if we are to prevent these severely ill people from living in flop houses, wandering streets with nowhere to go and nothing to do, being picked up and put in jails and just generally being seen by many as public nuisances. Many of these same people,

FOR THE EMOTIONAL AND SOCIAL PROBLEMS OF EVERYDAY LIVING

with treatment and supervised living and work environments, can be helped - even to the point of some productiveness and independent living.

Both you and I would rather for a member of our family or a close friend, if they were mentally ill, to be treated in Maury County Hospital and then they and their families be helped as outpatients than to be sent off to a state hospital or end up as a wasted life. J. B., we can steadily make things more like they should be in Tennessee if the Legislature will help get much more of the existing appropriation shifted over to the community mental health centers.

Bill Richardson has been keeping up with this and I know from our talks he wants to help the community centers. Senator John Hicks is providing some of the leadership in this direction. If you feel I can provide you with any information which will help in decisions on this complex matter, please let me know.

I am also enclosing a recent letter to Commissioner Sansom which presents an immediate concern related to a proposed shift of $3,000,000 for improving community services to the severely mentally ill. The share for the Columbia Area Center would be used to open a badly needed halfway house. Please do what you can to help us.

Sincerely,

George

George Spain, MSW
Executive Director

GS:df

cc: Senator Bill Richardson
Senator John Hicks
Mr. Dick Blackburn
Mr. Bill Walter
Mr. Doug Varney

(615) 388-6653

COLUMBIA AREA MENTAL HEALTH CENTER
OF CENTRAL TENNESSEE

TROTWOOD AVENUE
P. O. BOX 1197
COLUMBIA, TENNESSEE 38401

December 21, 1982

Senator John Hicks
5 Legislative Plaza
Nashville, Tennessee 37219

Re: Savings Resulting From Closure of State Institutes

Attention: Mr. Gene Russell

Dear Senator Hicks:

I continue to think about the meeting at your office on December 17, especially about the part relating to the % share which might go to community programs. While I have always thought that a portion of the State's appropriation to the Institutes would likely be "lost"to Mental Health, if one or more were closed, I have also believed it important that the major share go to community mental health centers. Originally the Department's formula for distribution of Institute savings was: 50% to community programs, 25% to the Commissioner for discretionary projects, and 25% for Institute improvements. As consideration is given to re-allocation of Institute appropriations, please keep in mind that:

1. Community Mental Health Centers have already assumed the ongoing responsibility for serving thousands of former "state" patients.
2. It costs us more each year just to maintain what we are presently doing.
3. These deinstitutionalized patients put a constant demand on local services and the pressure of sheer numbers has already shown us where gaps exist i.e. increased emergency services, the need for all kinds of community beds (hospital, crisis stabilization units, halfway house, boarding, independent living apartments and foster homes), more day treatment programs badly needed sheltered workshops, transportation, and more staff to do it all.
4. Seriously mentally ill children, adolescents, and young adults who once would have quickly gone into an Institute are also our responsibility as we try to treat them locally and prevent their ever getting into an Institute.
5. Community Mental Health Centers have many, many more responsibilities (others than the seriously mentally ill) that our communities and the state expect us to fulfill.

FOR THE EMOTIONAL AND SOCIAL PROBLEMS OF EVERYDAY LIVING

6. History evidences that those people who are both mentally ill and poor usually end up on the short end of the stick and we should do our best to prevent that happening. If Medicare and Medicaid benefits are reduced along with the federal grant cuts and all this is accompanied by closure of Institutes with only a minimal portion transferred to community programs the accumulative result will likely be a step backwards.

Because some mentally ill people are already not sufficiently cared for in their communities there are some prominent psychiatrists and others in Tennessee who feel we should now be using the Institutes more rather than less. If we fail in community care and treatment we may end up starting the cycle over again, back toward large institutional settings. Since none of us wants this to happen, it is essential that the legislature see to it that a major portion of state funds be transferred to the community if one or more Institutes are closed.

Sincerely,

George Spain

George Spain, MSW
Executive Director

GS:df

cc: Senator Bill Richardson
Mr. Dick Blackburn
Mr. Doug Varney
Mr. Chris Wyre
Mr. Wib Smith
Mr. Les Hutchinson
DR Bob Freeman

1982 WILLIAM F. ORR LECTURES

I first heard Dr. Orr lecture in 1959 when I was working on my Master's in Social Work. From then until now, he has been my teacher and professional role model. He is the high water mark by which I measure those of us who work in mental health. Years ago, one psychologist said of him, "He is not different in quality or quantity; he is different in kind." While definitely human, he exemplifies the best of what we are about. After my eight years of being in awe of him at Vanderbilt, I grew to love him during his four years as Director of the Mental Health Center at Columbia. I would hope for all the young clinicians here that you have, or will have, your Dr. Orr -- to stretch your thinking, to strengthen your courage to take a stand for what is right when it's needed, to increase your wisdom, to influence you to be practical, to help you care as much for the illiterate poor as for the highly educated wealthy, to retain the importance of your wife, children, and friends outside your work, and to see the importance of good humor and basic kindness.

Some of the things Dr. Orr enjoys are good literature, music, Chinese culture, museums, art, ballet and opera. Many of his patients were highly educated and well-to-do. At Vanderbilt, he worked with some of the best scientists and professionals in our nation. I have often heard him referred to as an aristocrat. Yet he came to help us in the country where most of our patients are poor and many have limited educations -- where the buck often stops with you and you may not have the readily available assistance and back-up of a large city.

He came to work in a Community Mental Health Center -- a system often criticized and doubted. He proved that community mental health can work and have a high degree of professionalism. And, when he retired his second time as Director, he left the foundation and standards for one of the best mental health centers in Tennessee. His standards remain and continue to influence our community, board, and staff, and are remembered by many of his patients. An example of his ability to explain, with very few words, a clear and correct standard for a complex problem was his quick response to my question, "How were mental health centers to avoid becoming what state hospitals became?" — "By keeping the focus on the needs of the individual."

To me, he has many qualities similar to Samuel Johnson, one of which Boswell gave in his "Life of Johnson," "His superiority over other learned men consisted chiefly in what may be called the art of thinking, the art of using his mind, a certain continual power of seizing the useful substance of all that he knew and exhibiting it in a clear and forceful manner," instantly relating one thing to another which helped him get to the point quickly and usually in a practical manner. So Dr. Orr clearly explains a complex dream or symptom by quotes from Freud and Charlotte's Web, Tolstoy and a limerick, Homer and one of his children, and it all hangs together and makes sense.

He considers the worst of all possible sins to be "ignorance rampant." While he does not suffer gladly those who should know better and behave foolishly, he is extremely kind and considerate. As Boswell said of Johnson, "His loud explosions were usually guns of distress." I well remember experiencing a few "loud explosions," but those were few and far between and only gave emphasis to his many kindnesses to me, his interest in my family and the sharing of our children's adventures.

We love to read his chart notes, filled with descriptions and observations which, in a few words, make the patient come alive. They show his interest in what some clinicians might consider small and unimportant things, but are of major importance to the patient and to understanding his life. They show his humanity, his intelligence, his honesty and wit, and the reason his patients love and respect him.

In one record, I followed the fortunes of a middle-aged, unmarried woman's cat (a Tom), who eventually went a-roaming never to return and was replaced by a new kitten. And there are suggestions of problems to come when he notes another woman had moved in with her dog. This dog was emphasized with an exclamation mark. And, in one of many letters of response to a bright young man with schizophrenia, who had colorful delusions and hallucinations, he wrote, "Certainly it is more fun to see a spade as a floating black bear (rather) than as a shovel, but it must be conceded that it is not as practical."

After retiring the third time from his job with the V.A. in New York, where he and Mrs. Orr went for a cultural sabbatical, they returned to Nashville. His eyesight prevented him from driving when he returned to Columbia as a volunteer psychiatrist, so two or three days a week he rode the Greyhound bus and became close friends with the bus driver. Among our staff, he remains a frequent reference point for understanding and serving the people who come to us for help.

To conclude, I will tell a personal experience we shared which exemplifies his fierce independence, occasional thunderous authority, wisdom, kindness, and courage to lose on something he believes in, for the benefit of someone he cares for: Our disagreement on salary for a social worker had gone on for some time and came to a head at a two-day planning session for Center expansion which was held at Paris Landing State Park. After a long day of planning, our intense debate/argument began that night and raged in color and sound, while the other three participants sat silent and white. Dr. Orr, as though he were confronting "ignorance rampant," asked, "George Spain, what is wrong with you? Haven't you learned yet that there is no justice in this world?" I replied, "Dad Blast it, I'm not talking about justice for the whole world, I'm talking about justice for her." Neither of us would bend or give way to the other. It hung in the air. Then, suddenly, he said, "Let's vote on it."

The vote hung on one person, as two of the other three were as though struck dumb and passed on their vote. Our Chief Psychologist voted my way. So I won and then what? Dr. Orr: "Let's get the bottles out and have a drink." He never referred to it again until I brought it up four years later while driving him home one night after it had been decided that I would take his place as Director. I recalled his once telling me that a Director should never allow the staff to make decisions by vote if the responsibility was ultimately that of the Director. I asked, "Why, then, did you suddenly call for a vote that night at Paris Landing?" Dr. Orr: "Because we were voting on something more important — our relationship."

It is such as this that makes him a great man and why he is always with me as teacher, guide and friend.

George Spain
September 23, 1982

COLUMBIA AREA MENTAL HEALTH CENTER
P.O. Box 1197, Trotwood Avenue
Columbia, Tennessee 38401
January 21, 1983

Dr. Karen Edwards
Tennessee Childrens Services Commission
James K. Polk Office Building
Suite 1600, 505 Deaderick Street
Nashville, Tennessee 37219

Dear Karen:

Damnit to hell, another boy has strangled himself to death with a bedsheet in a jail and he hadn't committed any crime! For God's sake this archaic treatment of putting non criminal young people in jails has got to be stopped. Because we continue to do it, the Trescott's son is dead. I believe all of us "responsible for helping young people, includ- ing pro- fessionals, legislators, Departments of State Govern- ment, Commis- sioners, and the administra- tion - past and present - bear part of the guilt.

While the Children and Youth Task Force report expresses con- cern about this, I fear, as with so many re- ports, nothing will be done. Can your off- ice take this on as a major goal? Since the big old state hospitals are probably on their way out, due to a lot of consist- ent and coop- erative effort, I believe the same could be accomplished on this. Minimal goals should be to make it against the law to put non criminal chil- dren in jail and emergency shelters should be made avail- able across the state.

Some re- sponsible group has got to stay angry about this and stay with it if we are to stop the troubled, but not criminal, children from tying sheets around their necks and strangling to death in a jail cell.

NASHVILLE BANNER
January 20, 1983

TENNESSEE SCENE

Runaway teen hangs himself in Marion jail

JASPER — A 17-year-old runaway from Ohio hanged himself with bedsheets while he was confined in a juvenile holding area at the Marion County Jail, according to Sheriff Loyd Hood.

Hood identified the victim as Ernest B. Trescott of Warren, Ohio.

Deputy Terry Parker said the youth had hanged himself from the shower head in his cell and was found Tuesday afternoon. The victim was the only prisoner in the juvenile holding area when he was found, officers said.

Sheriff's officers said they took the youth into custody Monday night at a restaurant in the Kimball community after receiving a complaint that he had been drinking and was disorderly.

Parker said a check of information shared through a nationwide police computer system showed that the youth had been reported as a runaway from Ohio.

Hood said Trescott had not been charged with anything and that he would have been released from the jail. Hood said the youth's family and Ohio authorities had not shown interest in coming to Tennessee to retrieve Trescott.

The Tennessee Bureau of Investigation is probing the circumstances of the youth's death, Hood said.

Yours sincerely,

George

George Spain, MSW
Executive Director

GS:df

(615) 388-6653

COLUMBIA AREA MENTAL HEALTH CENTER
OF CENTRAL TENNESSEE

TROTWOOD AVENUE
P. O. BOX 1197
COLUMBIA, TENNESSEE 38401

April 8, 1983

The Honorable John T. Bragg
33 Legislative Plaza
Nashville, Tennessee 37219

Dear Representative Bragg:

Chris Wyre speaks highly of your willingness to solve the problems that are occurring in the transfer of state funds from the Institutes to Community Mental Health Centers. It is now seven years since your 1976 House Resolution 400. The Centers are taking care of the majority of the severely mentally ill in their home communities yet almost 80% of the state's money remains with the Institutes.

In FY 1964 Tennessee had over 7,500 patients a day in the five Institutes. We are now down to less than 1,900 and it is my belief we can and should do considerably better.

I don't pretend to understand the complexities of difficult decisions and compromises involved in the total state budget during hard financial times - I do, however, see the patrol cars increasingly come to our Center for us to deal with a severely disturbed person. I do see some of the literally hundreds of patients who come to our eight clinics or psychiatric service at Maury County Hospital. Many if not most of these people would be in Middle Tennessee Mental Health Institute if we were not doing our job as expected. In 1962 our eight counties had 427 patients in State Institutes. Now we have less than 40. To do this we only get a little over $600,000 from the State.

Representative Bragg, the demands on us are beginning to tell. The Centers have got to have some big chunks of state money to take care of those very sick or handicapped patients.

Yesterday I attended your hearing of Commissioner Brown's budget presentation. I learned that a proposed $3,000,000 transfer to the Center's may be in jeopardy. With our Center's proposed share of $114,000 we are well along in the planning for a badly needed halfway house. With this we were hoping to drop our use of Middle Tennessee Mental Health Institute to 20 or less patients there a day.

It is like the Community Mental Health Centers had an agreement with the Department of Mental Health to build a new building and we were 3/4 finished

FOR THE EMOTIONAL AND SOCIAL PROBLEMS OF EVERYDAY LIVING

and weren't getting paid. Not only that, we are asked to add on some more rooms to the original house plan if we want to get some of our money. Or worse yet, we should take major responsibility for influencing their banker (F & A, the Legislature, the Tax Payers for a tax increase etc., etc.) to get them some money to pay us.

The Center's are doing their job and must have your help and that of Senator John Hicks and Senator Bill Richardson (he has been a long time supporter of our Center) to stop F & A from taking money away which could come to the community and to shift funds from the Institutes to the Centers. The fulfillment of the intent of House Resolution 400 is long overdue.

Help us get the $3,000,000 without it being dependent on a tax increase. Help us assure that, if the economy continues to improve, no more is taken away from the mental health appropriation. Help plan for responsible closure of two of the Institutes and transfer that money to the community. The patients are mostly out here now and we've got to have your help.

Sincerely,

George Spain

George Spain, MSW
Executive Director

GS:df

cc: Senator Bill Richardson
Senator John Hicks
Mr. Chris Wyre
Mr. Dick Blackburn

April 1983

TO: THE LEGISLATURE OF TENNESSEE

Your petitioners, Citizens of Maury County, respectfully petition the Legislature to enact legislation that will result in major reforms in the State's mental health appropriations and will enable improvements in community services for the severely mentally ill people of Tennessee.

On December 10, 1831, the people of Maury County petitioned your ancestors to help the mentally ill who were "confined in county jails" and "made inmates of Poor Houses." A copy of their successful petition is attached.

On October 19, 1832, the General Assembly enacted Chapter XXXI for the establishment of a hospital, "within or near the town of Nashville," for the care of the mentally ill. On a hillside, not far from where you now vote on the needs of our State, the first State Hospital opened in 1840. From this historical beginning, the State assumed and has maintained a major responsibility for the treatment and care of the mentally ill.

Now, one hundred and fifty-two years later, the people of Maury County return to the Legislature petitioning for major reforms in the State's appropriations for mental health services. While the majority of the mentally ill are now treated and cared for in the community, the major portion of state funding continues to go to the State Mental Health Institutes. Most of our mentally ill people have come home and, with regularly supervised care provided by Community Mental Health Centers, the number of patients in State Institutes has been greatly reduced. Twenty years ago, there were over 8,000 Tennesseans in our State and County Psychiatric Hospitals. Although our state population has since been increased by over a million people and we now have 2,000 or fewer patients in the five State Mental Health Institutes,

PETITION
TO: THE LEGISLATURE OF TENNESSEE

Page - 2 -
April 1983

almost eighty percent (80%) of the State's appropriation remains with these Institutes. State funds have not followed these patients as intended in 1979 (HB 1085) and 1976 (HJR 400). Our communities have received these fellow citizens back and accepted responsibility for their care and treatment. Now, all across our State they are in need of more medical treatment, hospital and residential beds, vocational and social training, sheltered workshops, day programs and help for their families. Your correction of this extreme imbalance in State funding will enable us to provide these most needed services.

We, therefore, petition the Legislature to enact such laws that will assure that a substantial portion of the State's funding for mental health services be transferred to Community Mental Health Centers. We further respectfully request that existing mental health funding not be reduced nor transferred to other Departments of State Government and that any funds received from the sale or lease of Institute lands or property be made available for the improvement or construction of community mental health center facilities. Lastly, we would suggest that provisions be made to assure that these funds go for services which are of direct help to those who are severely handicapped by mental illness.

We pray that you will respond as favorably to our petition as did your ancestors in the Legislature of 1831.

Respectfully submitted this _____
day of April 1983

PETITIONERS:

(615) 388-6653

COLUMBIA AREA MENTAL HEALTH CENTER
OF CENTRAL TENNESSEE

TROTWOOD AVENUE
P. O. BOX 1197
COLUMBIA, TENNESSEE 38401

August 2, 1983

James S. Brown, M.D.
Commissioner
Tennessee Department of Mental
  Health and Mental Retardation
James K. Polk State Office Building
505 Deaderick Street
Nashville, Tennessee 37219

SUBJECT: Formal protest of excessive forms and paperwork required of community mental health centers

Dear Commissioner Brown:

In a recent meeting of the majority of our staff, there was much discouragement and resentment expressed about the constant change in regulatory policies and standards which result in increasing documentation and a proliferation of forms. The general opinion of both clinical and administrative staff was that the completion of forms and other paperwork has reached the point of unreasonableness in trying to assure both the quality and quantity of our services and fiscal management.

This judgement comes from a mature, responsible and successful group of people who are well-trained and average eleven years experience in mental health, with six years at this Center. Their concerns, therefore, are not the irresponsible "gripes" often associated with complaints about "too much paperwork," but represent the serious judgement of mature and successful professionals. Needless to say, such feelings are one reason many good professionals do not seek employment in community mental health centers or leave centers for private practice.

As the top management officials of the Center, we cannot stand by and passively allow our fellow workers to become demoralized by feelings of futility and hopelessness. Because we respect them and concur with their concerns, we have a responsibility to find a solution which will help. What is our purpose? To provide care and treatment for the mentally ill and emotionally disturbed and to develop preventive programs. When paperwork and forms appear to be more important than the quality result of their work, we are defeating our purpose for being.

FOR THE EMOTIONAL AND SOCIAL PROBLEMS OF EVERYDAY LIVING

Commissioner James S. Brown
Tennessee Department of Mental Health Page - 2 -

Total trust of a person's word versus detailed documentation of all available, substantiating evidence are two extremes which require a reasonable, responsible balance. When the demand for detailed documentation begins to diminish the collective spirit of a group of responsible professionals, who have proven records of success, the line of reasonable balance has been crossed. When paper documentation becomes excessively institutionalized and is the ultimate measure of truth, it creates a conflict with the principles of trust which we promote and seek to achieve in our work with individuals, couples and families. In other words, we are not practicing among ourselves what we preach to others.

The appreciable amount of community support given to our Center and the communities' willingness to allow the severely mentally ill to return home and to remain here for treatment is based primarily on trust. This evidences that responsible accountability does not require excessive documentation.

We believe that certain documentation is essential for maintaining important history, supportive information, accuracy in decisions, planning, reliable and clear communication, accountability, and to assure substantive agreements. However, the trend toward increasing detail and expansion to more and more areas in order to prevent error and fraud is insidiously creeping beyond that necessary for responsible treatment and management.

Currently, as you will note in the enclosed list and individual copies, we have a total of 66 Forms which are required for clinical, fiscal and statistical recording. Recently, we spent considerable time and money revising our clinical records and forms to bring them in compliance with regulatory standards.

We respectfully request that the Department of Mental Health and Mental Retardation, with the help of front-line Center staff, initiate a study for the purpose of reducing, eliminating and consolidating records and forms now required of community mental health centers. We recommend that the development of new forms and reporting requirements be considered carefully by criteria similar to the following:

1. It is required by state or federal law, but does not exceed the intent of the law.

2. It will clearly result in better patient care or treatment.

3. It is absolutely essential to responsible fiscal management.

4. It is necessary for important research and future planning.

Commissioner James S. Brown
Tennessee Department of Mental Health — Page - 3 -

5. It will simplify, consolidate or eliminate existing form(s) and report(s).

6. The necessity for its use can be justified with substantial reasons which are not in conflict with other basic mental health principles and goals.

In conclusion, recall for a moment your work as a physician and consider the possible results that these forms might have had on your time and energy for treating patients. Would this accumulative detail have assured that you acted responsibly and made you a better physician? Would their collective total been necessary for the proper management and financial integrity of your office? Would they have increased cost to your practice and to your patients?

Only by translating these things down to the day-to-day realities of those who are actually providing care, treatment and management can we see the possibilities for end results that were never intended.

Surely, with your support, we can find some simpler ways to meet the requirements of accountability and thereby free up more time, energy and creativeness for helping people.

Sincerely,

George

George Spain, M.S.W.
Executive Director

R Barr

Ralph I. Barr, M.D.
Clinical Director

Danny R. King

Danny R. King
Business Manager

GS:RB:DK:bh

cc: Rick Sivley
Deputy Commissioner
Lee Fleisher
Assistant Commissioner
Robert Currie
Assistant Commissioner
Ben Dishman
Assistant Commissioner

Dick Blackburn, Executive Director
Tennessee Association of Mental Health Centers

COLUMBIA AREA MENTAL HEALTH CENTER

FORMS AS OF AUGUST 1983

LINICAL RECORDS AND FORMS

. Face Sheet
. Fee Evaluation
. Previous Record
. Initial Contact
. Patient Ledger Card
. Life Functioning/History
. Progress
. Discharge Summary
. Aftercare Plan
. Case Close Checkoff
. Substance Use
. Medical History
. Medication Profile
. Medication Log
. Medication Refill Form
. Treatment Plan
. Confidentiality Authorization
. A. & D. Abuse Questionnaire
. & D. Follow-up Letter
. ychological Examination
. Screening for Hospitalization
. Day Treatment Progress Inpatient
. Inpatient Social Services
. Transitional Services
. Emergency Commitment
. Judicial Commitment
. Voluntary Admission
. Inpatient Referral
. MIMHI - 30 Day Follow-up
. Utilization Review
. Day Treatment Scale
. Day Treatment Initial Plan
. Day Treatment Extended Plan
. Proposed New Legal Commitment Forms

STATISTICAL FORMS

1. Chronological
2. Direct Patient Service
3. Admission
4. Termination
5. Change in Status
6. CODAP Admission
7. CODAP Discharge
8. Client Flow Summary
9. 201 Card
10. 169 Statistical Summary
11. Clinician Time - Monthly
12. Personal Interviews
13. Collateral Visits
14. Staff Interviews
15. Boarding Home Modality Change
16. Day Care Modality Change
17. Inpatient Modality Change
18. Transfer Sheet
19. C. & E. Worksheet

FISCAL FORMS

1. Medicaid (11 pages)
2. State Budget (22 pages
3. Indigent Hospitalizati
4. Indigent Medication
5. Billing Form
6. Patient Receipt Form
7. Health Insurance Claim Form
8. Medicare Extended Payment Request
9. State Requisition
10. Local Requisition
11. Purchase Order
12. Travel Claim
13. Long Distance Telephon

*CAMHC 1983-84 Budget totaled 62 pages

Orr, 1st chief of VU psychiatry department, dies

Memorial services will be held Friday for Dr. William Frederick Orr, who became the first chairman of the Vanderbilt University School of Medicine Department of Psychiatry when the department was formed in 1947 and retired from the post in 1969.

Dr. Orr, 74, of 4706 Sewanee Road, died Monday in Graymere Nursing Center in Columbia after a short illness.

Memorial services will be held at 10:30 a.m. Friday at St. Ann's Episcopal Church. He donated his body to Vanderbilt Medical Center.

Upon retiring from Vanderbilt, Dr. Orr was director of the Columbia Area Mental Health Center until a second retirement in 1974, then a psychiatric consultant at Bronx Veterans Administration Hospital in New York, N.Y., until a third retirement in 1977.

He taught at Columbia University in New York, N.Y., and Harvard University in Cambridge, Mass., before joining the Vanderbilt University faculty in 1940.

Dr. Orr was born in Chattanooga but spent most of his childhood in Nashville. He was a son of the late William F. and Evelyn Fennell Orr. In 1941, he was married to the former Eunice Thompson.

He received his bachelor's, master's and medical degrees from Vanderbilt University.

Survivors besides his wife include two daughters, Miss Ophelia M. Orr, Boston, Mass., and Mrs.

Denver, Colo., John F. Orr, Chicago, Ill., and Merle T. Edwards-Orr, Burlington, Vt.; and six grandchildren.

Memorial contributions may be made to Vanderbilt University Libraries.

Nashville Banner, Wednesday, November 30, 1983 B-27

Dr. William Orr dies in Columbia

Memorial services will be held Friday for Dr. William Frederick Orr, who became the first chairman of the Vanderbilt University School of Medicine Department of Psychiatry when the department was formed in 1947 and retired from the post in 1969.

Dr. Orr, 74, of 4706 Sewanee Road, died Monday in Graymere Nursing Center in Columbia after a short illness.

Memorial services will be held at 10:30 a.m. Friday at St. Ann's Episcopal Church. He donated his body to Vanderbilt Medical Center.

Upon retiring from Vanderbilt, Dr. Orr was director of the Columbia Area Mental Health Center until a second retirement in 1974, then a psychiatric consultant at Bronx Veterans Administration Hospital in New York, N.Y., until a third retirement in 1977.

He taught at Columbia University in New York, N.Y., and Harvard University in Cambridge, Mass., before joining the Vanderbilt University faculty in 1940.

Dr. Orr was born in Chattanooga but spent most of his childhood in Nashville. He was a son of the late William F. and Evelyn Fennell Orr. In 1941, he was married to the former Eunice Thompson.

He received his bachelor's, master's and medical degrees from Vanderbilt University.

Survivors besides his wife include two daughters, Miss Ophelia M. Orr, Boston, Mass., and Mrs. Louise O. Comtois, Hooksett, N.H.; three sons, Dr. William F. Orr Jr., Denver, Colo., John F. Orr, Chicago, Ill., and Merle T. Edwards-Orr, Burlington, Vt.; and si grandchildren.

Memorial contributions may b made to Vanderbilt University Li braries.

Tribute to Dr. Orr, Mental Health Leader

EDITOR'S NOTE: Dr. William Frederick Orr died Monday at Graymere Nursing Home in Columbia. He served as director of the Columbia Area Mental Health Center from 1969-74 after retiring as the first chairman of the Department of Psychiatry at Vanderbilt University (1947-69.)

Prior to his tenure at Vanderbilt, Dr. Orr taught at Columbia University and Harvard University. He received his bachelor's, master's and medical degrees from Vanderbilt.

★★★

To the Editor:

I first heard Dr. Orr lecture in 1959 when I was working on my Master's in Social Work. From that time, he has been my teacher and professional role model. He is the high water mark by which I measure those of us who work in mental health. Years ago, a psychologist said of him, "He is not different in quality or quantity; he is different in kind." While definitely human, he exemplified the best of what we are about.

After my 8 years of being in awe of him at Vanderbilt, I grew to love him during his 4 years as Director of the Columbia Area Mental Health Center. He came to work in a community mental health center — a system often criticized and doubted in the early years — and proved that community mental health can work and have a high degree of professionalism. When he retired he left the foundation and standards for one of the best mental health centers in Tennessee. His standards remain and continue to influence our community, board, and staff, and are remembered by many of his patients.

He had many qualities similar to Samuel Johnson, one of which Boswell gives in his "Life of Johnson," "His superiority over other learned men consisted chiefly in what may be called the art of thinking, the art of using his mind, a certain continual power of seizing the useful substance of all that he knew and exhibiting it in a clear and forceful manner." So Dr. Orr could clearly explain a complex dream or symptom by quotes from Freud and Charlotte's Web, Tolstoy and a limerick, Homer and one of his children, and it all fit together and made sense.

Dr. Orr loved good literature, music, Chinese

and professionals in our nation. He was often referred to as an aristocrat, yet he came to help us in the rural areas where most of our patients are poor and many have limited educations. He once made the statement that he would "much rather smell the odor of good honest sweat than expensive perfume." His chart notes and reports are filled with descriptions and observations which make his former patients come alive. They show his interest in what some clinicians might consider small and unimportant things, but are of major importance to the patient and to understanding his life. They show his humanity, intelligence, honesty and wit, and the reason his patients loved and respected him.

I would hope for all young mental health clinicians to have their "Dr. Orr" — to stretch their thinking, to strengthen their courage to take a stand for what is right, to increase their wisdom, to influence them to be practical, to help them care as much for the illiterate poor as for the highly educated wealthy, and, lastly, to see the importance of good humor and basic kindness.

"You must always focus on the needs of the individual" is the professional standard by which Dr. Orr lived and it continues to influence the board and staff of this center. It is our greatest legacy.

— B. Spain

Opinions

'Former mental patient' use unfair

The following letter has been selected as the best of the week and the writer will receive $10.

By George Spain
1724 North Observatory Drive

Does the news media's periodic, but consistent, characterization of certain violent or disorderly people as "former mental patient" have some important implication for the public which I am missing? Is it just a continuation of what has always been done or is it considered truly newsworthy information that the community wants and needs to know?

I do not believe that studies clearly show a correlation between a wide range of mental illnesses and violence nor that a person who is mentally ill is prone to be more violent than anyone else. If it were so, the forever, ongoing debate on the ability of psychiatrists to predict dangerousness would not continue. I would like to suggest, however, that your management and editorial staff consider the possibility that the way "former mental patient" is continuously used may be hurting more people than you realize. It may play a part in maintaining old and false prejudices, stigmas and fears toward those people who have either brief or long periods of mental illness and who are no more violent than you or I.

If, however, "former mental patient" tells us something we really need or want to know then the scope should be broadened to include the rest of us when we "make the news." It could be argued, for instance, that this is relevant news information to include in news about people of prominence, whose daily decisions influence our entire community — people such as business and civic leaders, preachers, politicians, judges, physicians, lawyers, educators, psychologists and social workers.

On the other hand, if "former mental patient" is an attempt to show some evidence for cause and effect, might there not be other significant patterns that are being left out and should be made known to the public? For example, should we not include past, or present, religious, political, corporate, professional or civic affiliations on murderers, rapists, child abusers and thieves? Other "former" illnesses of the violator also might be significant. Who knows what will be uncovered? The possibilities are excitingly unlimited and would undoubtedly spice up the news and possibly increase sales.

I think we would all agree that these additional, ludicrous characterizations would be irresponsible and unfair to our fellow citizens and also to our "former mental patients." The description is inadequate and, in the long run, does undue harm to many people. The day may come when it hurts someone we love or even ourselves. It perpetuates a myth that fosters intolerance and rejection of those suffering from some form of mental illness.

If it does not conflict with fundamental integrity of the journalistic profession, I would appreciate your giving serious consideration to more discrimination, or the total elimination of the use of "former mental patient" when it is clearly not required.

Nashville Banner **FORUM** Friday, August 19, 1983

Editorials

Response to Mr. Spain's concerns

In the business of communications, and in the process of publishing newspapers in particular, practices which have come to be accepted for years continue to prevail, despite the fact that often they have become archaic and unfair.

A case in point has been brought to the attention of the *Nashville Banner* by George Spain, a Nashvillian with a career in mental health. Mr. Spain, in a letter which appears in the adjacent columns on this page, asks why the media continue to refer to people as "former mental patients" when such descriptions have little or no bearing on the story.

He has brought up a valid point, one which we are addressing, albeit belatedly. Identification of many people charged with committing crimes has too often been by the designation of "former mental patient," as if that bit of their life's history caused them to rob or steal or kill or evade the draft or whatever crime they may have perpetrated.

Why, then, have newspapers, including the *Banner*, continued to refer to "former mental patients"? We don't really know. We are taught in journalism school and in practice to use references in stories that have a direct bearing on the subject at hand. Using that logic, we would give a suspect's psychiatric history if he had committed a heinous crime and if we felt that history would help readers understand his actions. Similarly, when a man attempts to assassinate the president of the United States, it is not only fair, but a duty to report his background, including visits he may have made to a psychiatrist, because that may be traced to the behaviorial pattern that contributed to his crime.

In the Tuesday editions of the *Banner*, Ellen Therrien of the St. Bethelehem community in Montgomery County was referred to as having previously received treatment at a mental health center because we groped for answers in the death of her 20-month-old son. We felt readers, too, would seek answers, and so we quoted Clarksville police officials as saying she had received mental health treatment. We felt it was important to try to arrive at some understanding of her bizarre action and that it may have contributed to the murder of her baby boy.

We would not, of course, refer to a man assuming a corporate presidency or a businessman announcing staff promotions as a "former mental patient" because he may have visited a psyichiatrist at some time. Such reference would be out of place with the subject matter, but more than that, such a stigma would serve to inflict irreparable — and unnecessary — damage to their character and standing in the community.

As Mr. Spain correctly points out in his letter, studies have not shown a correlation between mental illness and violence, or that a person who is mentally ill is prone to be more violent than anyone else. Despite dramatic advances in the treatment and understanding of mental illness, psychiatric patients are often perceived as highly-disturbed, dangerous people.

Labeling a person as a "former mental patient" implies that his previous illness, which he may have suffered as a youth or 10 years ago, is the cause of whatever he may do or say or think. Illness of the mind, we know now, can be cured, as can illness of the body. We should not refer to past medical history in stories, unless that history has a direct bearing on the subject matter.

The *Banner* has routinely used "former mental patient" when that information was furnished by law enforcement agencies. But as a result of Mr. Spain's letter, and the concern he expressed that such unwarranted and unnecessary identification be subject to more discrimination or elimination of the use of "former mental patient" where it is not appropriate, we will take necessary measures to guard against its misuse.

The *Nashville Banner* has prided itself on being responsive to readers' suggestions and complaints. No communication to this newspaper from a reader goes unnoticed or unanswered. All are given careful attention. Mr. Spain's comments, however, struck a particularly responsive chord.

It quickly became apparent that his criticism was fully justified and in response, the *Banner* staff has decided to use identification that fits the story, particularly in cases of "former mental patient." With that decision, we cannot right wrongs committed in the past, but we can prevent recurrences in the future.

(615) 388-6653

COLUMBIA AREA MENTAL HEALTH CENTER
OF CENTRAL TENNESSEE

TROTWOOD AVENUE
P. O. BOX 1197
COLUMBIA, TENNESSEE 38401

August 24, 1983

Mr. Joe Worley
Managing Editor
The Nashville Banner
1100 Broadway
Nashville, Tennessee 37202

Dear Mr. Worley:

Thank you for the thoughtful and exceptionally well written editorial of August 19 on "former mental patients." Our staff appreciated your objectivity in considering our request and the openness of your presentation in the editorial response.

If other newspapers, radio and television stations were willing to follow your example, it could change some of the archaic beliefs about mental illness.

The management and editorial staff of The Nashville Banner are to be commended for their willingness to take the lead in helping to eliminate some of these old prejudices and stigmas about mental illness. Please convey my very sincere appreciation to Mr. Simpkins and others on your staff who contributed to the Banner's decision.

Sincerely,

George Spain

George Spain, M.S.W.
Executive Director

GS:bh

cc: Commissioner James Brown
Tennessee Dept. of Mental Health
Mr. David Moulder, Executive Director
Tennessee Mental Health Association
Mr. Dick Blackburn
Tennessee Association of Mental Health Centers

FOR THE EMOTIONAL AND SOCIAL PROBLEMS OF EVERYDAY LIVING

1983

George Spain
Executive Director
Columbia Area Mental Health Center
P. O. Box 1197
Columbia, TN 38401

Estimated Length: 4875

TENNESSEE'S MENTAL HEALTH SYSTEM

(A little bit of history and a whole lot of opinion)

by

George Spain

(With appreciation to
Dr. Robert Reed and
Dr. Ralph Barr for
advice and editing)

TENNESSEE'S MENTAL HEALTH SYSTEM

(A little bit of history and a whole lot of opinion)

* * * * *

It is a wet, cold Saturday morning in Nashville. I am waiting for the downtown public library to open. Outside the front door is a mixed bag of humanity: a few students; a nicely-dressed, middle-aged woman and her mother; an elderly couple; and several drably-dressed men who are sitting on the long, low walls beside the front door. All of these men appear to be poor. Some are unshaven and disheveled.

Now, as the doors are unlocked, I follow the wall sitters inside. They go in a beeline to sitting areas by the large windows of the main reading room. Here, they are screened from the librarian's desk. As I observe them more closely, it is clear that there are considerable differences among them. A few "old cronies" appear to be chronic alcoholics who have come here for warmth, sleep and the bathroom. Sitting by themselves are two young men who have received no recognition from the others. They may be transients. And, here and there, are individuals whose behavior catch my attention. They are neither noisy nor troublesome. One man mumbles to himself. The restless leg shifting and stiff posture of another resembles the side effects of prolixin, a medication used for treating schizophrenia. The expressions and actions of others suggest that they also are mentally ill.[1]

Who is to blame for mentally ill people wandering the streets of our large cities, often ending up in jails; sitting isolated in boarding homes

---

[1]The italicized inserts are this writer's memories of actual events which occurred at the Ben West Library and in two Tennessee psychiatric hospitals (one operated by the county, the other by the state). The first account is a composite of recent library visits. The second is from a 1940 hospital visit made when I was four years old. The others are from 1958 experiences as a social work student. While the emotional impact of these experiences and the warp of time may have created distortions, their essence remains true. It is even possible that the distortions are nearer the truth than I realize.

with nothing to do; remaining dependent on society because they have no job training, no sheltered workshops; becoming psychotic after stopping their medication and then being picked up by the police or sheriff's deputies? Who is to blame for the worry and anxiety placed on their families, friends, and neighbors? Who is to blame for the problems created for law enforcement, social agencies, hospital emergency rooms, community mental health programs? Who is to blame for these conditions unworthy of a state that prides itself on its institutions of health, religion and higher education?

A cautious answer might be that, in a democratic society, all of us share responsibility for the good and bad in our social institutions. The more straightforward answer is that the responsibility lies most with those of us who have direct influence on the operation and funding of statewide mental health services. This includes the Legislature, Administration, Department of Mental Health and Mental Retardation, Department of Finance and Administration, Tennessee Association of Mental Health Centers and the Tennessee Mental Health Association. They also deserve credit. In recent years major improvements have been made for people who have severe mental illness: better laws; accreditation of all five state hospitals; increases in state funding to community programs; and more local services.

We know problems exist and changes need to be made. But, as the proverbial blind men with their elephant, each of us touch only a piece of the problem and part of the solution. Like the blind men, we have difficulty agreeing on what we "see" as our future mental health system. As with the elephant, our system has been shaped by many influences. Both are big and complex. Yet, unlike our limited knowledge on how elephants were formed, we do know something about the development of our mental health system. Understanding a little bit of our history should be helpful in planning the future.

* * * * *

1840 - Tennessee's first hospital for the mentally ill opened in Nashville

1954 - Department of Mental Health established by Legislature
- 7300 patients a day in four state hospitals
- 4 mental health clinics operating

1964 - 7600 patients a day in five state hospitals
- 15 mental health centers operating

1984 - 1755 patients a day in five state hospitals
- 33 private, non-profit community mental health centers operating with over 85 county clinics.
- $75,376,200 appropriated by State for mental services (75% for state hospitals and administration, 25% for community mental health programs)

* * * * *

"Whereas, the great and increasing number of lunatics in this State, has made it necessary to the safety and well being of society, as well as for the comfort and security of these unfortunate beings, whom Providence has visited with the most severe of all earthly afflictions, that a suitable hospital should be erected in this State...."

- Tennessee State Legislature
October 19, 1832

Look again at that quotation from the 1832 legislative bill. Right there the priorities of concern are laid out with "the safety and well being of society" being assured before "the comfort and security of these unfortunate beings." This emphasis has continued to influence many decisions involving the mentally ill.

Before the first state hospital opened in 1840, it would be difficult for us to imagine the plight of the mentally ill. Even with the new hospital, Dorothea Dix's 1847 report to the legislature described the conditions still prevailing across Tennessee:

> "Were I to recount but briefly, a hundredth part of the shocking scenes of sorrow, suffering, abuse, and degradation to which I have been witness -- searched out in jails, in poorhouses, in pens and blockhouses, in dens and caves, in cages and cells, in dungeons and cellars; men and women in chains, frantic, bruised, lacerated, and debased -- your soul would grow sick at the horrid recital."

Because Miss Dix had committed her life to helping the mentally ill and had first-hand knowledge and experience of the conditions of that time, this great social reformer was able to sway the legislature to make major improvements. A 260-acre farm outside of Nashville was purchased and a larger and more accommodating hospital for the mentally ill was built on this site. It even had an apartment for Miss Dix in case she returned for a visit. The first hospital built in 1840 was called the Tennessee Lunatic Asylum. This new facility was named the Tennessee Hospital for the Insane, later known as Central State Psychiatric Hospital, and more recently Middle Tennessee Mental Health Institute. Though you can change a name, it is still true that as "a rose is a rose is a rose," so also a state hospital is a state hospital.

We are standing in a high-ceilinged lobby. I am between my mother and uncle. The lobby leads into a hallway which runs crossways to where we stand.

Passing in front, from our left, a guard, carrying a rifle over his shoulder in a military manner, strides down the hall, disappearing to our right.[1]

While Dorothea Dix's report influenced the changes made in 1852, they were also brought about by the increasing demands made of state government to deal with the social, health, and legal problems of an expanding population. Enlightened physicians contributed their support for better hospital care, although some continued to debate the merits of "bleeding" mentally ill patients. Some citizens, simply because of their religious and humanitarian beliefs, wanted the hospital to better the conditions of the mentally ill.

"Moral treatment" was the advanced practice of the time. This basically meant kindness, hygiene, nutrition, clean air, pleasant surroundings, comfortable buildings, recreation, constructive labor, and religious instruction for the mentally ill patient. These things were indeed beneficial and did help some people improve enough to return to their homes. For most, however, it was not sufficient.. There were major problems with moral treatment, including a scarcity of staff and programs to meet the needs of the patients. Since more people were being admitted than discharged, the results were overcrowded conditions and compounded problems. When you read those old yellowing superintendent's reports they sound very much like ones written a hundred years later — not enough staff, salaries too low to get well-trained people, old buildings in need of repair, new buildings needed because of overcrowding, more money needed from state government to provide better care and treatment. Year after year these reports, if one reads between the lines, tell of conditions which were unknowingly doing more harm than good for the mentally ill patients. Harm was not intended by the well-meaning and compassionate people providing these services, but as Dr. Robert Michels put it, "being a patient in a state hospital (was) more like having a disease than receiving a treatment."

Some woman keeps screaming. She breaks my concentration on the case record in which I write. As the screams continue, I wonder if someone is getting hurt. I rise, go out into the large hall and turn toward a heavy locked door. Carefully unlocking it, I listen through a crack. The screams are more piercing, but from where I stand I cannot see the woman. Locking the door behind me, I move slowly into the hall. There before me is a large wild-looking black woman twisting the arm of a small frail woman. I am reminded of someone wringing water from a towel. The frail woman screams and screams as I stand there, never having seen anything like this...[1]

Another big problem with moral treatment was that it did very little to treat the biological aspects of mental illness. Kindness, recreation and nice surroundings alone cannot reverse the changes in body chemistry which we now know contribute to such serious forms of mental illness as schizophrenia and manic depressive disorders. These disorders require medication, and it was not until the 1950's that modern chemotherapy began.

Most patients admitted after 1840 did <u>not</u> improve sufficiently to be discharged, and more and more people were being admitted from our rapidly growing population. Mentally ill patients were remaining in hospitals longer. Many of them were "forgotten" by their families. An increased dependence on the hospital as "home and family" became more the rule than the exception.

The hospital populations eventually resulted in five regional state institutes. The three oldest became larger than many towns in the state. By 1964 almost 7600 patients were being "kept" daily in the five hospitals, with almost 2500 in each of the three large ones.

Two white female aides close in on the arm twister -- one from the front to get her attention, the other, twisting a towel into the semblance of a rope, approaching from the rear. It is clear they know what they are doing. Their unhurried, easy methodicalness impresses me. In one smooth movement the rope-like towel is looped over the arm twister's neck. A few firm twists choke off her air supply and she falls to the floor, releasing her victim. I finally come alive and lift her legs as the aides hoist her up by her arms. We carry her into an iron-barred cell and lock the door.[1]

In 1942 Tennessee's first mental health clinic opened in Memphis. Because of new medicines, new laws and people speaking out about our treatment of the mentally ill, helpful changes began to occur. The state began to fund outpatient services which resulted in the establishment of new clinics. Twenty years after the Memphis clinic opened, fourteen clinics were scattered across the state. Their growth accelerated with the Community Mental Health Centers Acts of 1963 and 1965. Federal funds were provided to communities for the construction and staffing of community mental health centers. By 1976 combined funding from federal, state and local governments had resulted in our present thirty-three, private, non-profit centers.

With these developments the number of people in state hospitals gradually began to decrease. From a high of 7600 patients in the five state hospitals in 1964 there are now only 1755 patients on an average day. Another result was the closing of the old Davidson County Psychiatric Hospital in 1964. Until its closing over 600 patients were kept there daily. A line graph showing the decline of patients in state hospitals since 1964 resembles a slide moving closer and closer toward the ground. Where will it stop? Is it possible that within twenty years there will be no need for state mental hospitals? Once, all across America, there were county and state tuberculosis hospitals. Will our grandchildren remember that we once had state mental hospitals?

Some believe that "deinstitutionalization" -- the shift of treatment of the severely and chronically mentally ill from state hospitals to community programs -- has already gone too far. Some will point to those patients living in deplorable community conditions receiving little treatment and say that the shift has caused much harm. Some believe the need for state-controlled hospitals will continue indefinitely until other major advances are made in medical treatment. Others believe that the "death of the asylum" is at hand. Admitting that in some communities there are people who are underserved and living in terrible circumstances, they say that the majority released from our state hospitals have a less restrictive and a better life. They also say that community services would be markedly improved for all patients if community centers had a proper share of state funds. Seventy-five per cent, or more, of the state appropriation continues to go to state hospitals. The inequities in funding are shown in the following 1982 comparison of caseload and expenditures of state funds for the hospitals and community centers:

	Caseload*	%	State Expenditures	%
5 State Hospitals	11,876	12	$52,378,481	79
33 Community Mental Health Centers	84,690	88	14,048,858	21
TOTAL	96,566		$66,427,339	

*Caseload is number of patients on rolls at beginning of year plus all admissions during the year.

In recent years there have been rapid increases in local services for the severely and chronically mentally ill. Some community mental health centers are far enough along that, with a few additional programs, they would seldom have to use state hospitals to meet their patient needs (the single exception being those patients who have criminal charges against them). An example of this increased autonomy is the eight counties served by the Columbia Area Mental Health Center which once averaged over 420 people a day in state hospitals, and now average 34 or less.

There is nothing unique or sacred about state hospitals. They are just buildings with hallways, rooms, services and trained people who treat and care for patients with some form of emotional disturbance, mental illness, or brain impairment. Some argue that these hospitals provide services which cannot be made available at the same cost in the community. The cost of one bed for one year in a state hospital is over $35,000. Can communities not do a better job by putting this money in community hospital beds, residential programs and outpatient services?

On my first day I am taken on a tour of the two-storied building where I am to work for the summer. All the windows have heavy, strong screens. Many of the men and women have been here for twenty or thirty years. Many are never visited. One large smiling man dressed in overalls approaches me and begins telling me about the problems he has with his genitals. Throughout the summer he will recount this obsessive concern to me over and over. He is also excited about his upcoming visit home. I later learn that his family takes him home every year for a few weeks when the time comes to pick cotton.[1]

There is every reason to believe that medical treatment for the mentally ill will continue to improve. We have already come a long way from the years of moral treatment. Research indicates that chemical imbalances and genetic problems contribute to some of the more serious mental disorders. Mental illnesses are not all alike and their effects vary from individual to individual. Some may be long lasting while others are of short duration. Like diabetics who generally do well once their insulin dosage is stabilized, most people with mental illness can live responsibly and productively if they are treated with the right medication and receive professional counseling and social support on a regular basis.

Most of the middle-aged and older inmates of state hospitals have been discharged and are being successfully cared for in the community. We must now shift our attention to preventing admissions to state hospitals. Prevention will require more and better services for young adults at the time of their first severe symptoms. Many of their problems and needs are distinct from those of the older patient. They may be more demanding, harder to manage, less stable in living patterns and less reliable in following through with treatment. Along with their illness, they have the same difficulties as most in their late teens or early twenties: the conflict between independence and insolvency; the struggle in separating from parents; indecision about education and vocation; and the age-old conflicts of love, sex, alcohol and drugs. We tend to forget that most people who have mental illness are more like us than otherwise.

While touring the second floor men's ward, I glance into a bedroom to my left and something totally unexpected brings me to a halt. There beside his bed sits someone who is not supposed to be here. Only two years ago he and I had crossed the same stage, dressed in our black caps and gowns, to receive our college diplomas. Embarrassed, I manage to say something. He, maybe because he is sedated or because embarrassment no longer troubles him, handles the situation a lot better than I do...[1]

The success of community mental health programs may be determined by their ability to respond to the needs of young people. One negative influence of state hospitals on a young patient has been the tendency to foster dependency on an environment which provided for the individual's basic needs but required few decisions and little productive responsibility on the part of the individual. State hospitals have also provided a way to get the young, troublesome, mentally ill person out of sight and into a separate, controlled environment. Community hospital and residential programs will not provide the same degree of separation and control. While this difference may lead to some problems, it is important to establish therapeutic, yet socially responsible programs to serve these young patients and their families within their communities.

The time has come to consider another change in our state's 150 years of treatment for the mentally ill. The majority of mentally ill people are not dangerous. So why do we keep on using the police and sheriff's departments to transport patients? Law enforcement officers don't like doing it, but, more importantly, it is degrading and wrong to treat ill people in this manner. They are not criminals! They are ill! Surely a new statewide system under community mental health centers or ambulance services would be better since their emphasis is on health care rather than criminal control.

The majority of Tennessee's ninety-five counties now have outpatient mental health clinics operated by the thirty-three private, non-profit community mental health centers. While some areas of the state are farther along than others, none of these centers has yet reached a state of self-sufficiency in being able to totally care for its own. All across the state we need more local psychiatric hospital beds, crisis stabilization programs in residential settings, halfway houses, foster homes, long-term secure treatment facilities for the few who are violent because of their illness (but who are not criminals). We need more psychiatrists and other clinical professionals; social education services; outreach workers to make home visits and ensure follow-up care; vocational training; sheltered workshops; and better nighttime and emergency services. Development of these and other services will greatly improve care to those already discharged and living in the community. More patients will be able to leave the hospitals, and fewer will need to be admitted.

Both preschool and school-age children and their families are in great need of specialized community programs. The same is true for the elderly, those with alcohol or drug problems and the mentally retarded. While some of their needs may be met by present services, many more require specially trained clinicians and educators and specially designed programs and environments. Like the adult mentally ill they need more and better community programs to use in preference to state institutional services.

It is better for our families, friends and neighbors to be helped as near their homes as possible. It is better for a young person, when he has his first schizophrenic illness, to be treated in a way that fosters personal responsibility and independence. It is better for families to remain a part of the patient's life and treatment than to be separated by distances and restrictions. It is better to increase understanding and tolerance than to continue old prejudices. It is better for communities to meet their responsibility in caring for their own than to export the troublesome sick.

My classmate is still as shy, unassuming and quiet-voiced as he was in college. With polite certainty he tells me a rather strange story about a special message he received while listening to the preaching of one of our church's well-known missionaries. He seems unaware that the "special message" has ultimately led him to this room, to this building. The more he talks, the more I notice he already has the drab, unkempt, dull-gray appearance of those who have accepted this place as their permanent home.[1]

What prevents us from making major mental health reform in Tennessee? 150 years of history. Inertia to change. Personal dependency on the existing system. Political obligations. Lack of knowledge of what can be done to make it better. Fear of change, fear of added responsibility and fear of failure. Lack of commitment to help those who are often the hardest to help and may also be our poorest. Other priorities in state government and in communities. A lack of courage to confront those who control or influence the present system. The depersonalization of the mentally ill as though "they" are not like "us." Fear that if the state shifts further responsibilities to the community, the state will not shift state hospital funding to the community.

Lakeshore Mental Health Institute. Middle Tennessee Mental Health Institute. Western Mental Health Institute. The three oldest and largest of our state hospitals. Many of their old buildings still stand. Their halls echo with emptiness. Year upon year, money is poured into them for patching and propping where they crumble. Their broad fields, once filled with cattle and corn return to weeds and briars. Most of the people who once lived there have died or gone home.

Whether a decision is made to begin closing some of the hospitals or to keep all five open and reduce their size, two things must be fought for. No more state funding must be taken away from the mentally ill -- not for roads, not for prisons, not for schools, not for anything else! Savings at our state hospitals must go to help the mentally ill where they now live and need help — in the community. The same holds true for hospital lands and buildings. If they are leased or sold, the money must be retained and fairly distributed to build, buy or improve community buildings which serve the severely or chronically mentally ill. This land was purchased for them and now that they are being helped at home we have a continuing trust to use any funds received from these transactions to meet their needs for community hospital and residendial programs and for sheltered workshops.

It is vain to wait longer; to hope that those old buildings will fall down on their own; to believe that the practices of 150 years will be given up without conflict; to trust that reform will be initiated by the sheer weight of logic. It is already too late to retire from what must be done to make things better. Most of the mentally ill have come home. Our course and theirs are intertwined. They live with us, walk beside us, are our neighbors. They are no longer separate.

At the 1978 silver anniversary celebration of the Department of Mental Health and Mental Retardation, the former president of Meharry Medical College, Dr. Lloyd Elam, predicted: "I believe we will reach a point where we won't segregate our mentally ill and mentally retarded. We will recognize that they are us." Dr. Elam's prediction is already coming to pass. Each year, we "segregate (fewer of) our mentally ill." The more we help them, and they help us in the community, the more we "recognize that they are us." Now, the time has come for state government to shift it primary support from state hospitals to community programs!

In "The Death of the Asylum," author and psychiatrist Dr. John Talbott concludes: "I suspect that there will continue to be attempts at cosmetic change of the state mental hospital system, primarily in terms of changes in its functioning and roles. The times and economic pressures, however, will force society to scrap the system eventually because of its inability to solve the tasks assigned to it, and we will see the end of the asylum. The death of the asylum will repeat history, however, in that it will not provide a solution to the problem -- the treatment and care of the severely and chronically mentally ill. There will still need to be programs and services for this population -- including asylum-like settings. Whether this needed system will arise phoenix-like out of the ashes of the asylum or replace its death is problematic...Society will shuck off responsibility both for the state hospital system and the chronic mentally ill if given half a chance. We must not allow this to happen."

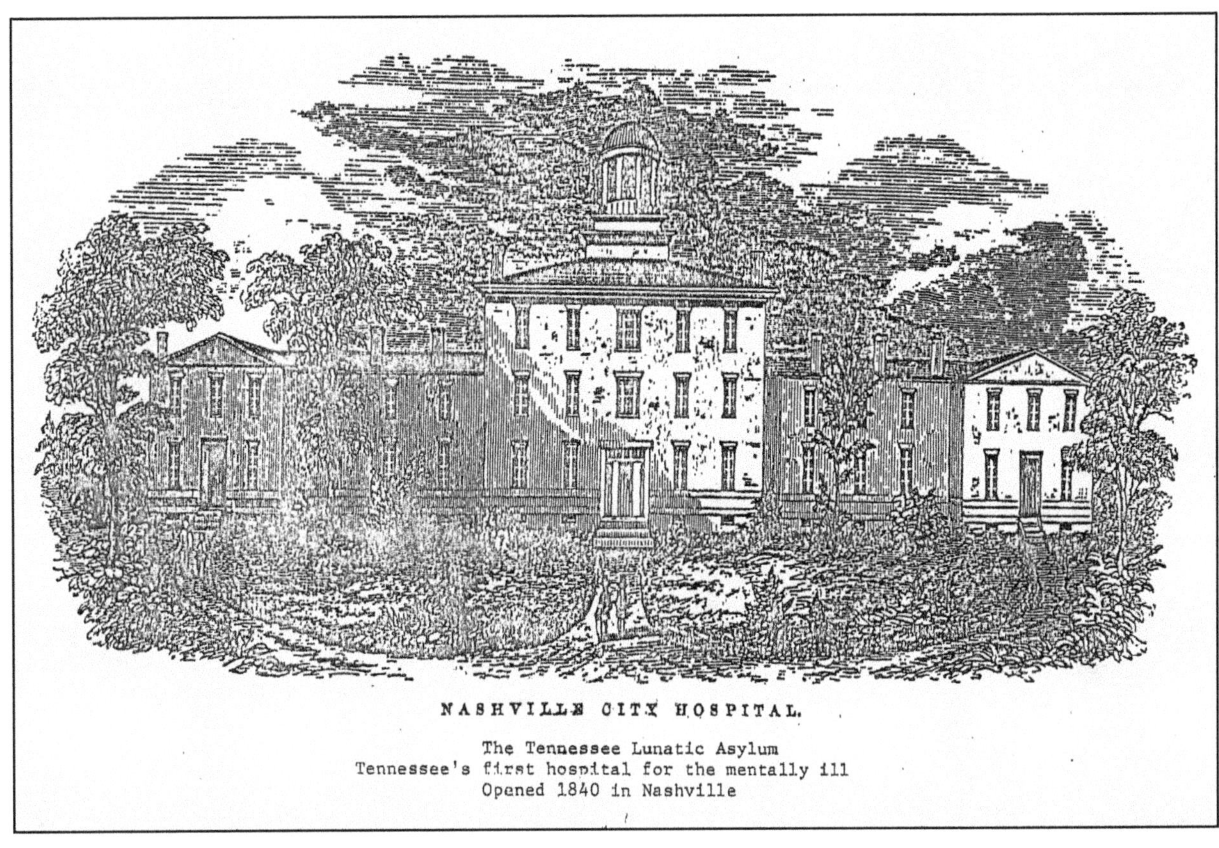

The Tennessee Lunatic Asylum
Tennessee's first hospital for the mentally ill
Opened 1840 in Nashville

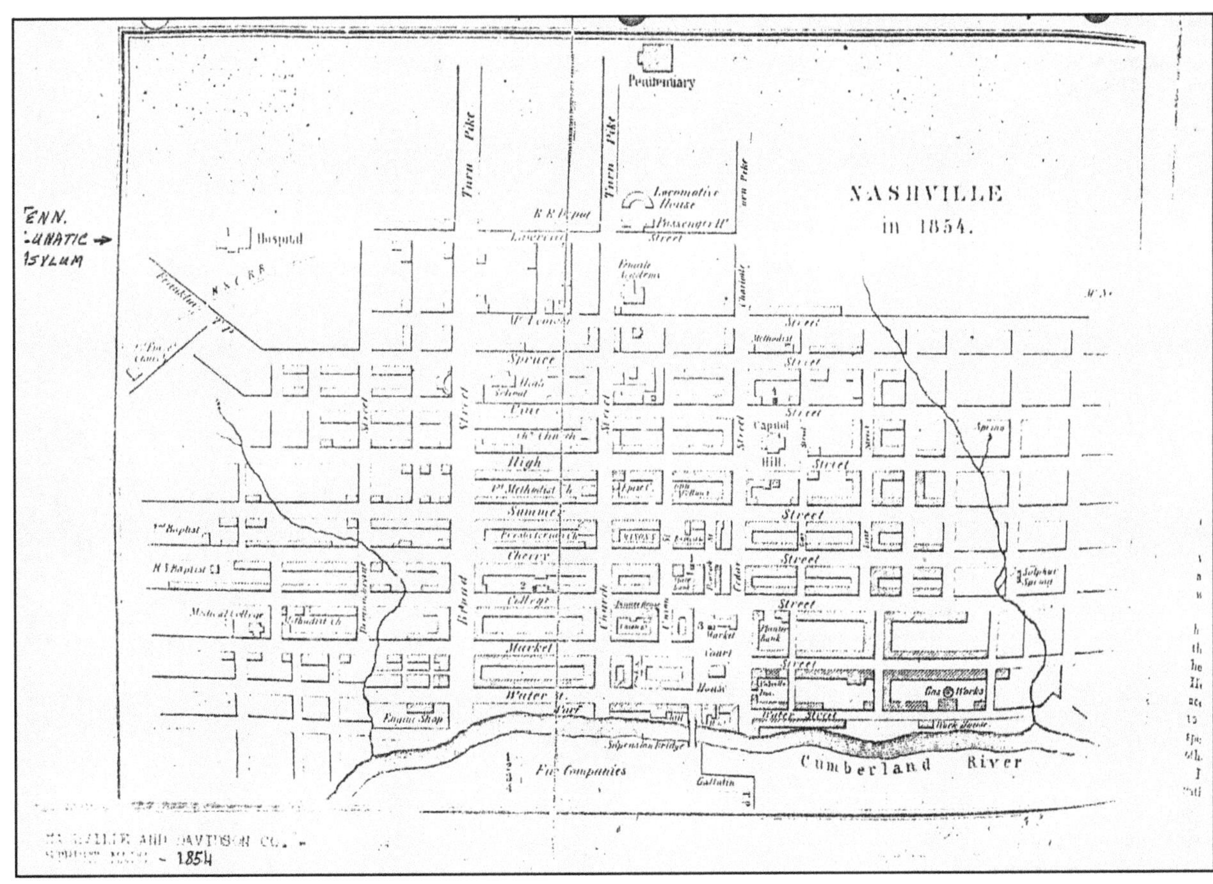

Nashville!

The Advantage Building
1719 West End Avenue
Nashville, TN 37203
(615) 329-1973

Atlanta:
Collinson, Holmes
& Associates
4315 Cowan Road
Tucker, GA 30084
(404) 939-8391

Midwest:
2 N. Riverside Dr.
Room 801
Chicago, IL 60606
(312) 930-9496

New England:
Catalyst Communications Inc.
244 Madison Avenue
New York, NY 10016
(212) 557-7510

Western U.S., Western Canada,
Mexico:
Zander and Bigler Inc.
6030 Wilshire Blvd.
Los Angeles, CA 90036
(213) 938-0111

22 Battery St.
San Francisco, CA 94111

Florida, Caribbean, South
America:
Coughlin/Adler Assoc. Inc.
Miami, FL 33156
(305) 665-1770

2950 Aloma Ave
Suite 201
Winter Park, FL 32792
(305) 677-4411

1/11/83

Dear Mr. Spain

Thank you so much for sharing this information with us. We are excited about the subject and plan to do an article this year on mental health in Nashville. At that time we will be in touch with you. Unfortunately, we can not use the material you submitted to us as it is. Grace Renshaw, associate editor of the magazine, will be in touch with you soon.

Sincerely,

Amy Lynch
Assistant Editor

An Advantage Publication

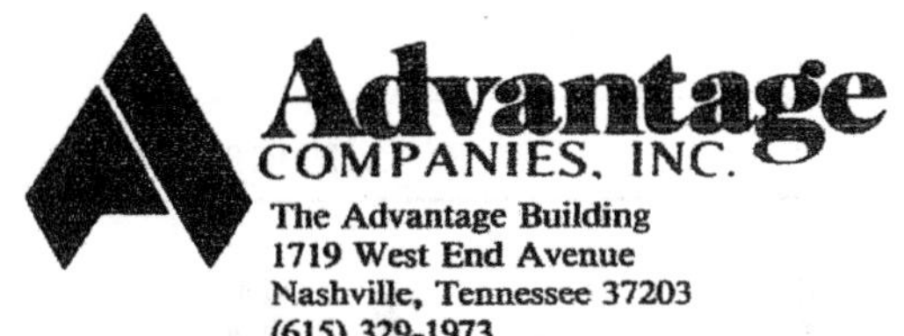

The Advantage Building
1719 West End Avenue
Nashville, Tennessee 37203
(615) 329-1973

January 11, 1984

Mr. George Spain, M.S.W.
Executive Director
Columbia Area Mental Health Center of Central Tennessee
P.O. Box 1197
Columbia, TN 38401

Dear Mr. Spain,

I read your article with interest, as the trend toward "deinstiutionalization" of the mentally ill, which has in some cases meant sending them back to families and communities that are ill equipped to handle their needs, had recently come to my attention as a possible feature topic.

I must tell you bluntly that we can't use your manuscript in the magazine. It contains too much editorializing and not enough information about the instutions and community centers that are now operating or the people they handle. I know in Texas, the Department of Mental Health and Mental Retardation publishes a newsletter for its employees; if there's a similar publication in Tennessee, your article would be ideal.

However, I am interested in covering the topic--with a special emphasis on the facilities in the Nashville area, and the families in the Nashville area who are coping with mentally ill members, along with the mentally ill who find themselves homeless or barely able to support themselves because of inadequate support from the state and their communities. I would be interested in using you as a source for this feature, and in printing some of your reminiscenses. (You would, of course, receive credit for them in print.) I might also be interested in editing your brief history of the evolution of mental health institutions into a sidebar (a short article that accompanies a major feature)--again, you would, of course, get a by-line for this piece.

If you are interested in acting as a source and a contributor, please get back with me.

Sincerely,

Grace Renshaw
Associate Editor, Nashville! Magazine

Publishes a DSM-III Just for

By Mary Ann Moon
Staff Writer

A Nashville psychiatric social worker has published his own guide to diagnosing psychiatric disorders, a spoof of DSM-III.

Besides giving readers a laugh, DSM (for Delightful Suthun Madnesses)-XIII (for the 13 confederate states) is meant to help mental health workers "retain a sense of humor about ourselves and face up to our own occasional ignorance," George Spain, the author, said in a telephone interview.

"In the kind of work we do, genuinely serious work where we have to make judgments about people's lives, we shouldn't take ourselves too seriously or get pompous," said Mr. Spain, executive director of the Columbia (Tenn.) Area Mental Health Center.

He denounces DSM-III as "a well-disguised commiepinkoliberal plot against beloved Suthun traditions," "a joke when it comes to diagnosing mad Suthunuhs," and "the ultimate of reconstructionist arrogance connived by carpetbagging Yankee eggheads."

The DSM-XIII uses descriptive terminology and illustrations by commercial artist Joe McClellan that Southerners can understand and appreciate.

"No longer will you have to use those ugly-sounding, Yankee diagnostic terms like 'dysthymia,' 'paranoid,' or 'anti-

Lobotomized Patients at High Risk for TD

International Medical News Service

WARD'S ISLAND, N.Y. — Patients who have undergone lobotomy are at high risk for developing severe tardive dyskinesia, and their neuroleptic therapy should be adjusted accordingly, say Dr. Carlos Leon-Andrade, of Manhattan Psychiatric Center, and his associates.

Of 94 inpatients with tardive dyskinesia, the disorder was more severe in those who had a lobotomy than in those who had not. This could not be attributed to differences between the two groups in age, sex, length of illness, or current neuroleptic therapy, the investigators say (Biol. Psychiatry 18:1329-1332, 1983).

Factors such as type of previous neuroleptic treatment, drug dosage, and serum levels may have contributed to increased severity of tardive dyskinesia in lobotomized patients, or the surgery may have heightened the brain's vulnerability to toxic effects of neuroleptics, the investigators say.

iatry News April, 1984

Southerners

social personality.' Your patients will know you are in sync with their problems when you tell them they have a bad case of 'the weary dismals,' 'narrow-between the eyes disorder' or 'mean as a snake personality,' " the DSM-XIII promotional literature says.

The DSM-XIII offers a compilation of homey descriptions for such maladies as "a mite bit tetched disorder" (these folks are "prone to unpredictableness, causing their kin and ole buddies to get a tad nervous when they come 'round; when you look deep into their eyes, they ain't always home"), and "highstacks" (hysterics), which, like "vapors" and "swimmy headiness," affect delicate Southern girls when they confront disagreeable realities.

Mr. Spain was inspired to compile DSM-XIII when he visited a boarding home for the mentally ill, where the director described a delusional patient as being "old and curious."

"I got to thinking, 'now, isn't that a nice way to put it, instead of calling it one of those things out of DSM-III.' "

He remembered several other down-home phrases that he had heard people use to describe behavior and decided to publish a list. Mr. Spain is no stranger to the publishing business, having poems published in Soviet Life magazine and Cumberland Poetry Review.

Mr. Spain, Mr. McClellan, and "an

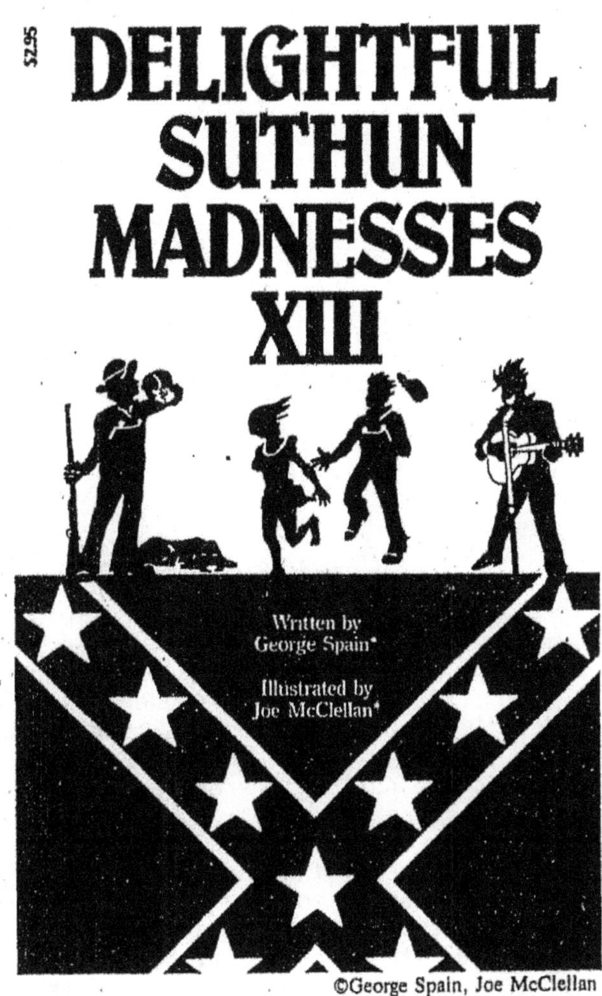

©George Spain, Joe McClellan

No, this isn't the latest DSM manual.

ole buddy" with a print shop intended to make 1,000 copies of DSM-XIII, but the stapler broke down at copy 827.

Meanwhile, Dr. Robert Spitzer, chairman of the task force that developed DSM-III, and chief of biometrics research at the New York State Psychiatric Institute, New York, said in a telephone interview that he is looking forward to studying DSM-XIII but reserves comment until he can read it.

(615) 388-6653

COLUMBIA AREA MENTAL HEALTH CENTER
OF CENTRAL TENNESSEE

TROTWOOD AVENUE
P. O. BOX 1197
COLUMBIA, TENNESSEE 38401

October 11, 1984

Doctor Nat Winston
Vice-President
Hospital Corporation of America
One Park Plaza
P. O. Box 550
Nashville, TN 37202-0550

Dear Nat:

Thank you for your support for an educational film on the historical evolution of Tennessee's beliefs about, and treatment of, the mentally ill. I believe there is an untold, fascinating story in this which would be both informative and entertaining for public educational television, high school and college students, civic and historical groups, mental health associations, boards of directors, and professionals. And, as you know, what has occurred in Tennessee is essentially what has happened across the nation; therefore, such a film has the potential for use in other states.

Since professional and social beliefs regarding mental illness (and the management and treatment resulting from these beliefs) are both an extension and shaper of general social values, it seems to me that the story would best be told in this mutually mirroring context. The viewer should see how our mental health beliefs and treatment reveal much about the ongoing evolution of society. Here, I think of the BBC series, Civilization, as a successful example. It portrayed and explained the development of western civilization "in its works of art, its buildings, books and great individuals." The sequences are greatly enhanced by filming the narrator, Kenneth Clark, in the presence of the actual building or work of art about which he is speaking.

As with Civilization, the film on mental health should include something on those individuals who have personified a particular event, or provided leadership in change -- such people as Felix Robertson, Dorothea Dix and Frank Clement. Interwoven to the main story would be vignettes that would add to the human interest and entertainment value of the film. For example, it might begin in Adams, Tennessee with a brief recounting of the Bell Witch, an event suggestive of

FOR THE EMOTIONAL AND SOCIAL PROBLEMS OF EVERYDAY LIVING

Dr. Nat Winston
Hospital Corporation of America Page - 2 -

medieval beliefs and fears of "unnatural" behavior. Then, there is Green Grimes who wrote two detailed and personal accounts in 1846 of his experiences as a mentally ill patient in the state's first hospital. Included in a list of the patients' diets was squirrel meat. Consideration was later given by the Legislature to turning this building into the governor's mansion. During the Civil War the effects of the Federal troop occupation of Central State Hospital are described with interesting detail in the superintendents' reports. The inclusion of such brief sketches, along with surviving pictures of buildings and artifacts, would add interest and help put the mental health theme in context with events of their particular time.

The move from the early 1800's management of the mentally ill in the community (poor houses, jails, lock-up rooms in homes) to the state hospital and now back to the community is a cycle that should be shown. The gradual shift from religious judgements, through moral treatment to Freud, and now into biochemical understanding of man's behavior should be evolved as the central theme. And, accompanying this, is the change from superstition and control to greater understanding and freedom for the mentally ill. The present problems of the homeless, chronically, mentally ill would also need to be shown.

Considerable research is needed to pull together the information that would be required by a professional script writer. The Department of Mental Health's soon-to-be-published The Development of Mental Handicap Policy in Tennessee (1796 to present) contains the skeleton of the history. What is needed, to give flesh, blood and life to it, are the words, actions and pictures of individuals, actual places and methods of treatment, with filming on sites that are representative of real events and real people. Add a good script, a professional film company, and a narrator who symbolizes Tennessee and a concern for helping others -- such as yourself, Johnny Cash, or Minnie Pearl -- and I believe it would be a film of considerable value for improving understanding and the treatment of the mentally ill.

I have spoken with Commissioner Sivley and he is responsive to the idea of supporting a film. Although the Department might not be able to offer financial support, they would cooperate in other ways such as offering staff assistance. The authors of the history mentioned above -- Paul Dokecki of Vanderbilt and Janice Mashburn of the Tennessee Department of Mental Health -- are also interested and willing to serve as consultants on this project.

We look forward to hearing from you about how we might approach H.C.A. Foundation for support of this project.

Sincerely,

George

George Spain, M.S.W.
Executive Director

GS:bh

(615) 388-6653

COLUMBIA AREA MENTAL HEALTH CENTER
OF CENTRAL TENNESSEE

TROTWOOD AVENUE
P. O. BOX 1197
COLUMBIA, TENNESSEE 38401

October 17, 1984

Mr. Richard D. Sivley
Commissioner
Tennessee Department of Mental Health
and Mental Retardation
James K. Polk Building
505 Deaderick Street
Nashville, TN 37219

Dear Rick:

Thank you for the opportunity to talk with you, Lee and Pam on October 9. I hope that I conveyed the strong concern felt by the center directors of Region V regarding state funding. We can no longer accept our region receiving the lowest per capita amount of funding, while maintaining the lowest use of the state institutes. What is happening to us is not the intent of House Resolution 400 (1976) and the 1979 Appropriation Act (Chapter 435 H.B. 1085). As the existing system is resulting in great inequity, it is our firm intent to seek a distribution policy which leads to regional equality of the total allocation and of the portion allotted to centers. While we realize that this cannot be achieved quickly, our experience is proof that it is not likely to ever occur unless it becomes a Department policy and thereby a major influence on annual budget decisions.

Years ago we joined with the State on the quest called "deinstitutionalization." In line with more recent goals, we have improved and expanded services to the seriously mentally ill. These goals and their accompanying service standards have been applied equally by the State to all centers and to all regions. Yet, Region V, with the lowest institute use, receives the lowest rate of funding. Need it be said that this is gross inconsistency and destructive to our incentive to do better.

Since Region V center directors and their communities bear responsibility for what is happening, it will not do for us to just complain about our situation, nor to later look back and say, "It was an accident over which we had no control." We are, therefore, determined to seek a policy of regional equalization which will result in true funding equity for all of Tennessee.

Mr. Richard D. Sivley
Commissioner
Tennessee Dept. of Mental Health   Page - 2 -

It is reasonable to anticipate that, with the exception of forensic inpatient services, the day is coming when private providers will assume total responsibility for Tennessee's mental health services. That is the ultimate extension of what has been developing over many years. Coupling this with the fact that the majority of the mentally ill are now cared for by community programs (and the realistic clinical potential for caring for many more, if not all, in the community), then: <u>a long range policy that provides for an equal, regional distribution of total state funding is essential.</u>

Regional equalization would not prevent community programs, in one or more regions, from receiving a greater proportion of funding needed in a given year to establish major costly services. It would mean, however, that in subsequent years other regions would be prioritized and provided the same support, all within the ultimate goal of an equal distribution of the total appropriation.

Without a long range policy governing total funding, it is reasonable to expect that:

1) Inequity of funding will continue on, as it has from one Administration to the next;

2) Community services for the mentally ill will continue their erratic development across the state;

3) Community providers will be hampered by the absence of a fixed, long range framework within which to plan the development of services;

4) The interminable "every man for himself" attempts at obtaining special deals with the Department will continue; and

5) The state legislature could become involved.

It is clear from the recent figures prepared by the Department that the present funding distribution of centers and regions is resulting, at best, in considerable inequity and, at worse, in extreme inequality. Equal funding of regions is consistent with the following beliefs:

1) Large regional populations are relatively equal in their mental health needs.

2) Regional equality of funding supports the development of equal distribution of services.

3) Future advances in medical/social treatment of mental illness will result in community programs assuming greater responsibility and thereby further diminish the need for state institutes.

Mr. Richard D. Sivley
Commissioner
Tennessee Dept. of Mental Health   Page - 3 -

4) Political/societal shift toward government decentralization will continue.

5) Understanding and acceptance of mental illness will continue to improve so that individuals, families and communities will prefer services provided as near their home as possible.

6) A clear funding framework for the total appropriation enables an orderly and fair distribution of state funding.

7) The present funding system prolongs historical inequities and emphasis on institute utilization which are in conflict with present and future shifts to community treatment.

This Administration has sufficient time left in the remaining two years to set in motion a regional, equal funding process that prepares for, and supports, the above beliefs.

Region V has well proven its commitment to serving the severely mentally ill. We have been patient on the inequality of state funding. Now, our patience has run out as we bear the responsibility of our success in helping the Department accomplish its goals. We are now requesting that the Department and the Tennessee Association of Mental Health Centers give priority attention to developing a plan which results in equality of regional funding. We agree that our cooperative solution is much to be preferred over the involvement of the state legislature.

Sincerely,

George

George Spain, M.S.W.
Executive Director

GS:bh

cc: Region V Center Directors

Dick Blackburn, Executive Director
Tennessee Association of Mental Health Centers

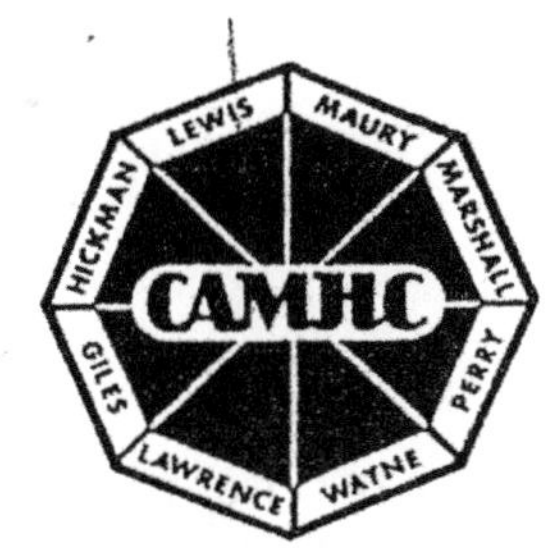

MEMORANDUM

TO: Community Mental Health Center Directors

FROM: George Spain GS

DATE: November 6, 1985

RE: CMHCs Establishing Services in Columbia Center Service Area

As there is a growing belief that there should be no geographical limitations on a center's developing non state-funded services in another center's area, let me make my personal position absolutely clear. If any center, combination of centers, or their subsidary, or their cooperative venture with another corporation, attempts to establish a service within our area without involving Columbia in the initial considerations, there is going to be hell to pay!

Just so there is no confusion on the area we serve, it includes the counties of Giles, Hickman, Lawrence, Lewis, Marshall, Maury, Perry, and Wayne.

GS:df

COLUMBIA AREA MENTAL HEALTH CENTER
P.O. BOX 1197, Columbia, Tennessee 38402-1197 Telephone 615/388-6653

STATEMENT TO BOARD OF DIRECTORS
TENNESSEE ASSOCIATION OF MENTAL HEALTH CENTERS
March 27, 1986

"Lest I be criticized for hypocricy and for acting holier than thou, let me first admit that I personally learned a painful lesson over two years ago. It was that the lust of extreme selfishness results in behavior that is flagrantly stupid, dishonorable, and wrong.

Yesterday, after our meeting, I learned from Glen Burse that Health Services Initiative, Inc., a subsidiary of Quinco Mental Health Center, has opened an office in Columbia. I first heard of this when one of our staff met Barry Hale, Executive Director of Health Services. Quinco's behavior has, for some time, created distrust and conflict in region six and now it is spreading to other areas.

The belief that anything goes in the struggle for survival, or to achieve one's ambitions, is apparently held by others in this Association. At our last annual conference the Meharry director learned inadvertently that Dede Wallace had plans for setting up a day care center in Meharry's service area.

Glen told me that he wasn't even sure Health Services Initiative was still under Quinco or him. Here clearly, is one of the destructive symptoms of expansionism, that it exceeds one's good judgment and ability to manage. We are not first industries, we are not first big businesses - - we are first mental health centers and should practice what we preach to couples and families - - clear communication, trust, and honesty.

You all can debate this thing until hell freezes over, while the ties of this Association are hurt or even torn assumder by the disregard of some for basic courtesy and integrity. I will not wait for you!

I therefore, publically censure Quinco Mental Health Center for creating distrust and conflict in region six and for spreading it to region five. And, I will inform Glen's board of his actions and ask if they condone them, and if they do not, what action do they plan to take".

Presented by: George Spain

GS:df

PRESENTATION TO THE MENTAL HEALTH STUDY COMMITTEE SJR 161 TENNESSEE LEGISLATURE

December 2, 1987

Members of the Legislature, Ladies and Gentlemen. In the past, it has been rare that people with mental illness speak out at a public forum such as this about their needs or their ideas about the way things can be made better. I hope, and believe, that some will tomorrow. What they say should be carefully listened to.

There are, however, many of us as providers of services who, from our different perspectives, want to speak for the needs of the mentally ill in Tennessee and for those who have severe emotional problems, for the children, adolescents, the adults and the elderly. For those who have schizophrenia or a manic-depressive disorder, or who are incapacitated by depression or anxiety, children with autism and those who have been abused or neglected. And for the mentally ill and terribly depressed old people who live alone or in nursing homes. The mentally ill wandering our streets. And those who feel so hopeless they want to kill themselves, as a friend of mine recently did. And for their families who want to help, and can help, but who may need a boost themselves, or better understanding of what the illness does, and what they should do.

And, finally, I'm here to speak for our state's non-profit community mental health centers who have pulled in harness with the state for a long, long time -- beginning in a small way almost forty years ago. We have worked hard at eliminating the warehousing of people, far from their families, and often forgotten. We have succeeded in building a statewide system of clinics within a short distance of home for anyone needing mental health services.

Let me begin with some personal history. I am a native Tennessean and have lived here all my life. For thirty years. I have worked with people who have mental illness. Tennessee has come a long way in those three decades and, all in all, I believe we have done a fair and decent job. One of my two earliest memories, before I was five years old. is of a mental hospital -- the old Davidson County Psychiatric Hospital, closed in the mid-sixties. I was there with my mother and uncle visiting his wife. Eighteen years later, I trained and worked there a year. During the next year, I had a summer job at Central State and worked with patients who had been there twenty and thirty years and who were seldom, if ever, visited by anyone. After graduating, I worked eight years in the first child psychiatry inpatient unit in the south, at Vanderbilt -- which state funding helped support. And then in 1967, I went to work at the Columbia Area Mental Health Center and have been there for twenty years. Our eight-county service area had almost 430 people in the state hospitals twenty-five years ago -- now we average thirty.

The Department of Mental Health and anti-psychotic medications were still new when I began working. While there were approximately one million fewer Tennesseans then there were over 8,000 patients in the four state hospitals and Davidson County Psychiatric Hospital. There were eleven (11) mental health center located in nine (9) counties.

Today, while our population nears five million, we now average only 1600 patients in the five state hospitals. Davidson County, which once held over 700 patients (more than are presently in any one of our state hospitals) closed down its psychiatric treatment twenty years ago. We now have thirty-two mental health centers, with clinics operating in ninety of our ninety-five counties. In 1986, these centers' combined case-loads neared 90,000, with one-third being patients for whom state funding has been prioritized because of the severity of their problem.

While last year we celebrated Homecoming Tennessee, the mentally ill have been coming home for a long time. In many ways, much is better for people with mental illness. They are not packed away in old buildings, locked away and forgotten, far from their families and homes. Their legal rights are better protected. Medical care has generally improved. The length of psychosis and need for hospitalization is shorter. Our community services are steadily evolving better programs to meet their needs. Thousands of Tennesseans have served on community boards where they have gained knowledge and understanding of mental illness and, in turn, educated their friends, neighbors and relatives, thereby decreasing prejudice and stigma.

<u>But</u> we all know much has not been done and needs doing. A few blocks from here, on Broad, ranging from Union Station to the river, are some people wandering the streets and alleys

who are mentally ill. Nearer here, at the Ben West Public Library, right now, there are probably a few mentally ill people sitting in the reading section back of the stacks. And, in smaller institutions called boarding and nursing homes, all across our state, there are mentally ill people who are at dead-end streets. You already know of their plight for community housing, residential treatment programs, and crisis stabilization units. A recently completed Department of Mental Health study projects a need for more than 2,000 community beds for housing and treatment. Many, many more case managers are needed to help them, and their families, obtain the services that are available.

We are doing a lousy job, next to nothing, when it comes to vocational rehabilitation and sheltered workshops. We need to continue to expand preschool programs such as R.I.P. and the therapeutic nurseries which have proven successful in helping abused and neglected children, as well as those with autism, developmental delays, and severe behavior problems. We have just begun to set up programs for adolescents, but these are few and far between. There is little to no statewide leadership nor funding to develop special community mental health services for the elderly who are mentally ill. They, most likely, are our most underserved people. We need more people with special training to help children, adolescents, and the elderly.

Most of the mentally ill live among us and most prefer it that way and most do better by being helped near their homes. Yet, still, most of the state's money for services (70% of it) goes to state hospitals. Quite frankly, that is not the way it should be. And that is one thing the Legislature should direct the Department to correct, but it should not be done by cutting institute funding, but by increasing appropriations, over time, to community progra

Now, for some recommendations:

1) The first is basic and general. Build upon that which exists and has proven its commitment and its success -- non-profit community mental health centers. I have known and worked with six Commissioners of Mental Health since 1965: Dr. Nat Winston, Dr. Frank Luton, Dr. Richard Treadway, Dr. Harold Jordan, Dr. Jim Brown, and Rick Sivley. With all their differences, they have all been advocates for building a strong, statewide system of non-profit community mental health services. And, my assumption is that Commissioner Eric Taylor so believes and will do likewise. Yet, from time to time, we hear rumors of putting community mental health services out for bids, as we do with roads and buildings. People who advocate this either know little about severe mental illness or their focus is more on business and money than on care and treatment. Think for a moment about yearly or bi-yearly bidding out of community services to the low bidder and its potential for changing locations, providers and routines. Then consider the confusion of thinking, the difficulty in trusting, and the anxiety and fear that often occurs with mental illness. Stability, continuity, familiarity, and trust developed over time with a particular person or group of people is often essential to someone agreeing to take the medicine or guidance that is offered. So, the Legislature could do a lot by a

resolution recommitting itself to the non-profit community mental health providers who have worked with you and the Department for several decades to build the foundation of our existing system. As part of this resolution, we and the Department need support for a bold and multi-yeared push that emphasizes community services such as we had in the Community Initiative Plans from 1983-86.

2) There should be a codification of per capita funding of community mental health centers so that all communities can be assured of a strong, basic level of support, no matter what changes occur in the Administration or Department. This will help assure the maintenance of a basic level of services across the state. It should be noted that the major, severe mental illness, schizophrenia, occurs fairly consistently amongst us, whether we are poor or rich, city or country-bred, black or white. In 1975, I heard a legislative budget committee take Dr. Jordan to task for the extreme inequities that existed in funding from one community to another. As a result, the Legislature spoke out clearly for establishing a level of fairness across the state in House Resolution 400 which was signed by Speaker of the House Ned R. McWherter. It read:

> "WHEREAS, there appear to be inequities in the distribution of state appropriations to community mental health centers and community mental retardation programs across the state: now, therefore,
>
> BE IT RESOLVED BY THE HOUSE OF REPRESENTATIVES OF THE

EIGHTY-NINTH GENERAL ASSEMBLY OF THE STATE OF TENNESSEE, THE SENATE CONCURRING, That the department of mental health and mental retardation be directed to study the needs and determine the method for distribution of funds to community mental health centers and community mental retardation programs in Tennessee so that per capita equity and local effort may be established."

3) During the past year, a great deal of time has been spent by the Department and Centers on establishing new licensure requirements for community programs. Concern continues to exist that the proposed requirements are excessive and that more time and work should be given to reducing them to only those that are absolutely essential. Excessive licensing requirements reduces funds and staff time for direct services. We are requesting clarification of the legislatures intent relative to TCA 33-2-501, the licensure law, and a study of the fiscal impact of the proposed rules on contract agencies

4) Community programs serving the mentally ill, and those with severe emotional problems, need more funding to improve existing care and treatment, and to expand such services as case management, supervised housing, residential treatment, crisis stabilization units, vocational services and specialized programs for children, adolescents, and the elderly. Severe mental illness is long-lasting and costly and many people have no third party coverage.

- Medicaid should be expanded to cover those who may work, but have low incomes. Medicaid should not however be seen as the sole panacea for funding, as it is directed at medically approved services and cannot be used for other needs. It may get you medicine, hospital care, and day treatment, but it doesn't help on housing, transportation, case management, job training and sheltered workshops.

- Vocational rehabilitation funds should be made more directly accessible to mental health service providers. The existing Vocational Rehabilitation system has inherent conflicts in trying to serve motivated physically handicapped and mentally retarded clients in comparison to those with mental illness whose energy, motivation, and goals may fluctuate and be totally disrupted due to their illness. I have heard that our state has turned back unused federal Vocational Rehabilitation funds. If true, it should distress us all and should be rectified in the future.

- State appropriations should be increased and new dollars directed to community programs where the majority of the mentally ill are served. The existing proportion of 30 percent to community programs and 70 percent to institutes should be directed, according to a time-limited schedule, to move toward a 50/50 split.

- Tennessee has started a big push to build community services for children and adolescents -- partly influenced by the goal to deinstitutionalize delinquents. Community mental health centers are expected to play a major part in this through service on the Interdepartmental Case Assessment Management (ICAM) and with evaluations and other services. Yet few additional funds have come to the Centers to cover this cost. Needless to say, we cannot pull our manpower out of one deinstitutionalization battle and put them in another and expect to do either well. I, therefore, recommend that you approve S1,250,000 to hire 32 full-time psychological examiners who will work full-time on ICAM evaluations and related mental health services for this new effort.

- And last. In 1848, your predecessors authorized a commission to establish a new hospital for the mentally ill, "for the care and safekeeping of at least 200 persons." This led to the state buying a 255 acre farm six miles out on Murfreesboro Road. The new hospital, 320 feet long, 50 feet wide, with 138 rooms, opened on April 19, 1852. To most of us, it is known as Central State Hospital -- though officially as Middle Tennessee Mental Health Institute. In the 1960's, 110 years after it opened, it held over 2500 patients -- 900 more than all five hospitals across the state hold today.
  As you know, the three older hospitals -- Central, Eastern State, and Western -- are large in buildings and lands in comparison to Memphis and Moccasin Bend. At these older hospitals, the mentally ill were housed and treated, and were provided employment where they raised their food and sold the surplus. Now, most of the mentally ill are gone from these hospitals and are living among us -- too

often without proper housing and most often with no employment. At Central State, most of the land stands idle, its weeds and briars housing and feeding only rabbits and starlings. For 140 years, the land has been there as a long standing trust for the care and safekeeping of the mentally ill. It is a trust that was long-maintained, but, in recent years, piece by piece by piece, it is being lost forever and one day it can all be gone. We must protect what is left. We must adapt the original purposes to fulfill present day needs. I am, therefore, asking your support for SB 1194 and HB 1174 (Bill Richardson and Ben West, Jr.) either in its existing form which would result in the sale of unused lands or for an amended version, preferred by Governor McWherter, which would allow for long-term leasing of these unused lands. The revenue would be put in a trust fund which would be used for no interest or low interest loans to build or renovate community facilities that serve the severely mentally ill. The fund should be used solely for the mentally ill and should be fairly distributed to both rural and urban communities. Funds for the mentally retarded should likewise come from any state developmental centers where unused land exist. This revenue should not go to the General Fund, nor should it be used for the purpose of decreasing other funds or appropriations. It is hoped this legislation could become law quickly, or, until it passes, that some legislative restraint be initiated which would prevent one more acre from being lost. Without additional taxes, and without losing the state's capital, the Legislature has, with these unused lands, an untapped resource to improve community care for the mentally ill.

In preparing for this, I came across a part of Governor Clement's presentation when the Department of Mental Health was founded in 1953. It is appropriate to what this Legislative Committee seeks to accomplish:

> "This means a higher standard of care, a more specialized type of supervision a more humane approach to the problem of mental illness, and, above all, a greater opportunity for the mentally ill to be returned to their homes and loved ones."

Working together, we have come a fair way toward meeting these expectations. Hopefully, this Committee will provide new expectations and influence toward future improvements for the mentally ill.

George Spain, A.C.S.W.
President
Tennessee Association of
Mental Health Centers
December 2, 1987

MEMORANDUM

TO: Executive Committee, TAMHC
Legislative Committee, TAMHC

FROM: Dick Blackburn
George Spain G Spain

DATE: January 23, 1987

RE: Use of Excess Mental Health Institute Property

I initiated this + it became law - I count it one of my best achievements G. 2009

The Legislature's first appropriation was $10,000 on October 19, 1832 for land purchase and construction of Tennessee's first mental hospital. Subsequent Legislatures increased appropriations for improvements and to add new hospitals, reaching our present number of five state hospitals in 1962. A review of early legislative reports and bills evidence that both the lands and buildings were for the ongoing care and treatment of the mentally ill.

The Legislature's commitment to helping the mentally ill now dates back in an unbroken line for 155 years. While the extent of legislative concern has waxed and waned over the years, the consistency and growth of state funded support evidences a clear intent of responsibility, especially for the indigent.

The high in total state hospitals patient census was in 1963 -- 7500. Since then, due to new laws, new medicines and community care, the number has steadily declined toward the present 1500. Since community programs now provide most of the care and treatment, there are major needs all across Tennessee for housing and vocational and treatment facilities. The likelihood of the Legislature approving substantial new money for community capital projects is probably zilch. For that reason, we should gain their support for a plan which results in a legislative bill which:

1. Recognizes that the care of the seriously mentally ill who are indigent has mostly shifted to community programs.
2. Recognizes that there are major capital funding needs in both urban and rural communities to renovate or construct new facilities for housing, vocational training and treatment.
3. Provides for an updated study of the five mental health institutes' lands to determine how much unused property is available (see TDMHMR Response to Chapter 755 of the Public Acts 1982, p. 39 and TDMHMR 1988-1991 Four-Year Plan, p. 96.)
4. Provides for the sale of the unused property and the placing of all the income into a trust fund which is used for low interest loans on non-profit community capital projects which serve the indigent, seriously and chronically mentally ill. (I understand that the legal rule of cy-pres should be used to support this proposal and that these may be helpful in Tennessee case decisions and legislative precedents.)
5. Provides for equitable distribution to urban and rural communities.

I would suggest that we get our lobbyist's reactions and recommendations to this proposal. Consideration should be given to working on this in collaboration with the Department and various volunteer advocacy groups.

Senate Bill No. 1642

by

Richardson

1/20/88

H/B 1507 Wes

AN ACT relative to certain property of the department of mental health and mental retardation, and to amend Tennessee Code Annotated, Title 33.

BE IT ENACTED BY THE GENERAL ASSEMBLY OF THE STATE OF TENNESSEE:

SECTION 1. All property owned or held by the department of mental health and mental retardation which is not in use shall be sold or leased in accordance with the provisions of Tennessee Code Annotated, Title 12, Chapter 2, Part 1. The procedures for selling or leasing such property shall begin to be implemented immediately upon the effective date of this act.

SECTION 2.

(a) Notwithstanding the provisions of Tennessee Code Annotated, Section 12-2-112(7), the proceeds received from the sale or lease of such land shall be deposited in a special trust fund created by Section 3 of this act.

(b) The revenue earned from such trust shall be used by the department of mental health and mental retardation for the development of mental health or mental retardation community facilities, depending on whether the property sold or leased was a portion of the grounds of a developmental center for the mentally retarded or a mental health institute. Trust earnings generated by funds from the sale or lease of developmental center property shall be used for capital improvements, such as construction of facilities, housing, or other nonprogrammatic uses, benefiting the mentally retarded. Trust earnings generated by funds from

11410234 14162C

the sale or lease of institute property shall be used for capital improvements, such as construction of facilities, housing, or other nonprogrammatic uses, benefiting the mentally ill.

(c) The corpus from such trust may be used for the purposes provided in subsection (b) as provided in regulations promulgated by the department.

SECTION 3.

(a) There is hereby created within the general fund a special trust fund earmarked for the sole purpose of generating revenue to provide funds to the department of mental health and mental retardation in the development of mental health and mental retardation community facilities as provided in Section 2 of this act.

(b) Proceeds from the sale or leasing of the property owned or held by the department of mental health and mental retardation which is not in use, pursuant to Section 1 of this act, shall be deposited in such special trust fund. Provided that funds in such special trust fund shall be consolidated with state funds under the control of the treasurer in the same manner and as provided in Section 9-4-704.

(c) Interest accruing on investments and deposits of such fund shall be returned to the fund and remain a part of the fund.

(d) Any unencumbered funds and any unexpended balance of this fund remaining at the end of any fiscal year shall not revert to the general fund, but shall be carried forward until expended in accordance with the provisions of this act.

(e) Except as provided in subsection (b) of this section for administration expenses, all funds in the account and interest earned from such funds shall be used for the purposes provided in Section 2 of this act. The state treasurer shall have the authority to promulgate necessary and appropriate rules and regulations to implement the effect

-˙- 14162C

and intent of this section in accordance with the Uniform Administrative Procedures Act, Title 4, Chapter 5.

SECTION 4. The department of mental health and mental retardation shall promulgate rules and regulations in accordance with the Uniform Administrative Procedures Act, Title 4, Chapter 5, relative to utilizing the corpus of such special trust fund and relative to separating and accounting for the funds within the special trust fund pursuant to subsection (b) of Section 2.

SECTION 5. This act shall take effect upon becoming a law, the public welfare requiring it.

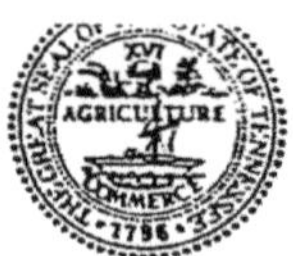

State of Tennessee

HOUSE BILL NO. 2433

By Representatives Wood, Johnson, Halteman, West, Severance, Coffey, Odom, Ruth Robinson, Walley, Clark, Brenda Turner, Callicott, Nuber, Larry Turner, Kent, King, Hubbard, Pruitt, Fowlkes, Tullos, Knight, Hargrove, Meyer

Substituted for: Senate Bill No. 2561

By Senators Crutchfield, Atchley, Albright

AN ACT relative to certain property of the Department of Mental Health and Mental Retardation, and to amend Tennessee Code Annotated, Titles 12 and 33.

BE IT ENACTED BY THE GENERAL ASSEMBLY OF THE STATE OF TENNESSEE:

SECTION 1. Tennessee Code Annotated, Title 12, Chapter 2, Part 1, is amended by adding Sections 2 through 5 in this act as new, appropriately designated sections.

SECTION 2. All property owned or held by the mental health institutes enumerated in Section 33-2-101 and controlled by the Department of Mental Health and Mental Retardation which is not in use may be sold or leased in accordance with the provisions of this part. The procedures for selling or leasing such property shall be those required by law and the State Building Commission for other state owned real property.

SECTION 3.

(a) Notwithstanding the provisions of Tennessee Code Annotated, Section 12-2-112(7), the proceeds received from the sale or lease of such land shall be deposited in a special trust fund created by Section 4 of this act.

(b) The interest and principal from such trust shall be used as provided in the general appropriations act for the specific purposes of planning and construction of mental health facilities as well as for the transition of patients from an institutional setting into community programs.

SECTION 4. There is hereby created within the general fund a special trust fund earmarked for the sole purpose of providing funds to the Department of Mental Health and Mental Retardation for the purposes set forth in Section 3(b).

SECTION 5. The Department of Mental Health and Mental Retardation shall not submit a budget that proposes to use funds derived from the sale or lease of property owned or held by the department to supplant its current level of appropriated funding.

SECTION 6. This act shall take effect on July 1, 1992, the public welfare requiring it, and shall not apply to any land sale initiated prior to July 1, 1992.

This was passed by the Legislature 1992

TESTIMONY PRESENTED BY GEORGE SPAIN, TAMHC PRESIDENT,
TO THE SJR366 LEGISLATIVE STUDY COMMITTEE
OCTOBER 19, 1988

Mr. Chairman and members of the Committee thank you for staying with the work of making improvements in our state's mental health services system. The severely mentally ill and their families need more help and services than are presently available. All of us know that. At the top of all our lists are housing, case management, psychosocial programs, public education, vocational rehabilitation, and, whenever possible, work.

There is much, much good in the Department's plan -- especially as it identifies needs and services to help the severely mentally ill. The Department is to be commended for its energy, for its bringing together of a lot of people with varied views, but with a common concern to make things better for those with mental illness. Those of us who have spent time with Joyce Judge, Ray Signor, and Bob Long know they have influenced our thinking about the needs of the mentally ill and their families. Clearly, we can make, we _must_ make some greater commitments.

Our concerns and disagreements with the plan are these:

1) While community mental health centers have a major and a primary responsibility for treating and caring for the severely mentally ill, we have also been expected, and rightfully so, to help others who suffer from severe emotional disorders and less severe mental illnesses. In finding ways to better help the severely mentally ill, we must not abandon these other people, many of whom are the working poor, who without insurance or State subsidized funding, will have nowhere to go -- that just would not be right. These people suffer and hurt like people with schizophrenia and bipolar disorders. Let me tell you who they are. (Here Mr. Spain read excerpts from a letter written by Debbie Adkins, a member of the Tennessee Mental Health Consumers Association, which is attached.)

   In the audience today is Debbie Adkins, a member of the Tennessee Mental Health Consumers Association from Morristown. She states in a letter written to Bob Waters, Director of Planning and Evaluation, DMHMR, that her main concern with the Department's plan is in regard to "potential targeting of mental health funding for a very limited population of mental health consumers." She then points to the kind of symptoms a new patient would need to exhibit to qualify for State subsidized services. "It is unreasonable to expect people to suffer to such an extent before making services avaiable to them," Ms. Adkins stated in her letter.

(Mr. Spain then pointed out other people in need who would not qualify as priority population.)

Emotional [illegible]

- A friend who had committed suicide and left a husband and two teenage sons.
- An abused wife in Maury County.
- Survivors of the Maury County jail fire.
- Farm families experiencing financial crises.
- Robertson and Sumner County families who are having loved ones exhumed due to illegal practices of a funeral home operator there.

The Study Committee, in presenting its recommendations last year, recognized the need to continue to provide services to these non-priority people who have insufficient financial support. They need to have you stick with them.

2) There is little to nothing said about the needs of our State hospitals.

3) The plan recommends the establishment of a single mental health entity (authority) in Davidson County. This entity, as described once to us, would be put in place over the four existing community mental health center boards -- in essence, another layer of bureaucracy. (How much will it cost and who will pay for it?) Time and again we have expressly opposed this in regional and state meetings, yet the Department continues to pursue it. Please give this up -- it is not needed to do the job. Listen to such better ideas and ways as presented by Region II -- the use of interagency compacts and agreements, a proposal supported by the centers <u>and</u> the advocacy groups. Under the heading of <u>Problems Encountered by People Who are Mentally Ill</u>, page 3.2, there are two incorrect statements: (Mr. Spain read excerpts from the plan and made brief comments.) "There is no single State entity that has the authority to coordinate and distribute all the resources available to provide for the needs of the mentally ill."

4) Reference to [illegible] concerns about former dept. person and funding chgs gaining a foot & possibility some centers could be hurt

But there is. It is called the Tennessee Department of Mental Health and Mental Retardation.

"There is no single entity on the local level that has the recognized responsibility or the care and treatment of the mentally ill."

But there is, there are thirty-one community mental health centers with responsibility or those who live in their respective catchment areas.

Do not support these unnecessary changes and risk the loss of community boards and their help.

4) There are profound funding changes being proposed by Medicaid and the State. Much of their stated purpose is to improve accountability and targeting of funds. I have said it til I'm blue in the face -- take care, take care! Nothing should be done that significantly changes the balance achieved over many, many years. You remember how all that State money was going to follow the patient from the State hospitals to the community? Well, once we had almost 8,000 in the hospitals and now there are 1600 and most of the money went back to the general fund. So we scratched and shifted and learned ways to make it work. And all in all, the money is well spent. While there are still inequities in funding communities, much improvement has been made. Since 1985 community mental health has received no improvement funding and even lost $2 million in FY1988. We need to focus more on improving services and on obtaining reasonable increases that are fairly distributed across the State and that are used for targeted services -- as we did with Community Initiative funding. AND ONE MORE TIME, let me say it is a sin, a crime, and a shame that we are not getting use out of the unused State institute lands. They should be sold or leased and the funds put in a trust fund to use for such things as badly needed housing for the mentally ill, which the Department estimates would require $40,000,000. Why in heavens sake do we not put those weeds to work for us out on Murfreesboro Road? I have Senator Richardson's bill and a bill from California that tells how it can be done.

The mental health centers have learned a lot in the past year during our meetings with consumers and families. Positive changes are occurring by our talking and working together. The Tennessee Association of Mental Health Centers must be with them in their advocacy for improving services for the severely mentally ill, but we cannot do this exclusively as we are also looked to for help by others who suffer. What we seek is reasonable and responsible balance. As Tennessee has no single inspired person like Dorothea Dix, Clifford Beers, or Frank Clement that everyone sits up and listens to as a champion for all those with mental health problems, it falls to us collectively -- the Legislature, the Governor, the Department of Mental Health, the advocacy groups, and the providers to work together as their champion.

SPEECH TO TENNESSEE MENTAL HEALTH ADVOCATES

STATE CAPITOL
MARCH 22, 1994

Three years ago, I had a cancer cut out of my chest. If it does not return I may be cured, and I will die of something else.

When I was a boy, the dreaded disease for children was polio. If you got it, you died or ended up with braces and canes. Jonas Salk developed a vaccine, and now, polio is prevented.

But if, when I was eighteen, I had started having jumbled thoughts, and heard voices directing me to act in certain ways, and begun to behave in ways that disturbed and even frightened my family and friends, I would have been hospitalized and probably diagnosed as having schizophrenia. So would have begun a lifetime of being treated with medications and hospitalization and receiving support from various community services. And, today, I would stand before you still having schizophrenia, still requiring help. And, I would go to my grave with that illness.

Severe mental illness is in many, many ways different from physical illnesses. As yet, there is no prevention, there is no cure. There is only control of the symptoms. With medication, counseling and support services there is the good probability of living with a fair degree of independence, and productiveness and, living with more hope in the community.

There is still no prevention, there is still no cure. People with mental illness have special needs, and because they still face prejudice, they still require champions. Today, here in this House Chamber, you who have come from the great Smokies in the east to the great Mississippi in the west, from the big cities and from the country, you, today, are their champions.

In 1831, one hundred and sixty three years ago, this was written: "To the Legislature of Tennessee. Your petitioners, citizens of Tennessee, desire that you.....appropriate a portion of the [new] Penitentiary House for the comfortable keeping of the Lunatics of our State...some are confined in county jails, others are made inmates of Poor Houses. It occurs to your petitioners that suitable apartments could be made as a sort of Hospital.....allowing the Lunatics to be under the care and attention of the regular physicians....."

This petition of 146 Tennesseeans led to the legislature appropriating the first money to help the mentally ill and to the building of the State's first hospital in 1840 -- within one mile of this Capitol.

Seven years later, in 1847, the greatest champion this nation has ever had for the mentally ill, a one time school teacher, Miss Dorothea Dix, came to Tennessee to investigate the conditions of the mentally ill. They were deplorable. Still in jails and poor houses, still chained, or wandering at large. She wrote a magnificent memorial to the legislature, entitled: For the Insane Of the State of Tennessee. Because women could not address the legislature, it was read by a man. It resulted in the purchase of a large farm and the building of a modern and well conceived hospital -- now known as Middle Tennessee Mental Health Institute.

Within this very building, the next historical landmark occurred. March 13, 1953 (only forty-one years ago) Frank G. Clement, Governor of Tennessee, signed the legislation which created the Department of Mental Health. He had also found deplorable conditions in the care of the mentally ill and believed that the creation of a separate cabinet level department was essential to the improvement of their treatment. In Lebanon, in 1954, he said, "I hope that someday the opening paragraph of a Tennessee history yet to be written will say of my administration [that], the aged, the needy, the lame and the halt, the blind and the mentally ill citizens were the first beneficiaries of unprecedented recognition and advancement".

Right from the beginning, the Department of Mental Health conceived that an integral part of its mission was the return of the mentally ill from the state hospitals to the community, and that, with local financial support and cooperation, people could be treated within their community and "be restored to society with the least possible permanent impairment".

Beginning in 1955, funding was set aside in the budget for the establishment and support of community clinics, and, by mid-1957, our four large cities had them. From the first, down until now, this mission has continued as a partnership between the State and the Community.

In April, 1983, in the State Senate, another petition was read. It refers to the 1960's when the five state hospitals and one county hospital held more than eight thousand mentally ill Tennesseans. But now it says: "Most of our mentally ill people have come home and, with regularly supervised care provided by Community Mental Health Centers, the number of patients in State Institutes has been greatly reduced to fewer than 2,000.....Our communities have received their fellow citizens back and accepted responsibility for their care and treatment." The petition then requests "that existing mental health funding not be reduced nor transferred to other Departments of the Government", but be used for community services where most of the mentally ill were already being served. By the end of the 1980's, practically every county had its own clinic.

And now we come to the present. The hospitals have steadily declined in size, and the community services have increased. Under federal regulation, and with first class leadership from the Department of Mental Health, and with the support of our legislators, we developed one of the finest mental health plans in the nation - Tennessee's Master Plan. This plan was developed with the help of hundreds of people, some with mental illness, some family members and others, advocates and providers. Now, slightly over mid way along, community service and care has been improving in quantum leaps. Things for the most part, not conceived of ten years ago, are provided all across the state: Intensive case management, psycho-social rehabilitation programs, mobile crisis teams, community housing, supported employment, drop-in centers, community support teams. Together the partnership between state and community had designed a Master Plan which is working in increasing independence, hope, and better conditions for the mentally ill. But, it is not complete!

Now, here we are today, suddenly and unexpectedly, in the throes of TennCare, which, with all its good financial intentions and desire to make things better in health care, has within its present structure the potential for doing serious harm to mental health services and the Master Plan.

Because TennCare was underfunded, suddenly the decision was made to take state and federal funds for mental health and put them into TennCare -- over $300,000,000 that would have gone specifically for the care and treatment of the mentally ill is now within TennCare. No longer ear-marked for the mentally ill, significant portions of these funds could end up being used to pay for physical care -- even for such things as hernias, ulcers, and kidney stones. Unless these funds are kept separated for the mentally ill, they can be steadily eaten away, for, as Frank Clement realized, the mentally ill will not get the attention required for their special needs unless the funds and decisions regarding their use are separate from physical care. A way to do this must be found within TennCare.

All the Master Plan's social support services could be lost under the present Managed Care Organizations which give no recognition nor payment to these essential services. These services will gradually disintegrate and ultimately disappear. And if that happens, where will the mentally ill go? Thousands, upon thousands, upon thousands, of state hospital beds are gone. Where will they go? Back to the jails. To the poor houses of our day - the Union Rescue Missions. More and more wandering again as in Dorothea Dix's day - homeless. We will slide backwards, backwards, toward 1953, 1847 and 1831. And after awhile, the community will say enough, and somewhere, out in time, we, or others, will have to start over to rebuild what has been lost. What a tragedy!

In short, TennCare must be changed in a manner that does not harm its responsible and rightful goals, yet finds a way to clearly separate those funds necessary to assuring the achievement of the Master Plan. Funding must be clearly designated for the care and treatment of the mentally ill. This must be done!

Think of all those who have gone before us, all those champions for the mentally ill, those 146 in 1831, Dorothea Dix and Frank Clement, governors, and legislators, commissioners of mental health, hospital superintendents, psychiatrists and social workers, counselors, psychologists and nurses, the Department's Board of Trustees and thousands of volunteer community Boards of Directors, and all the legions of the mentally ill and their families. Think of their presence around us. Think of all they have achieved. And then think, how can we do less? How can we go backwards in time? We cannot!

Now, our time here ends. It is time to go out to talk with our legislators - to convince them to find a way within TennCare to separate funds specifically for services for mentally ill adults and children. Today, is our day to be champions for the mentally ill.

BY: George Spain, Executive Director
Columbia Area Mental Health Center

AMENDMENT NO. House #260
Of the Appropriation Bill

FILED
Date
Time
Clerk
Comm. Amdt.

Signature of Sponsor

AMEND Senate Bill No. 2820 **House Bill No.** 2760

by adding the following new item at the end of Section 10:

Item ___. The commissioner of health shall calculate the total amount of funds for mental health services based on (a) the amount of funds that the bureau of medicaid and the department of mental health and mental retardation budgeted, as of December 31, 1993, for (1) those mental health services that are now covered by TennCare benefits and (2) administrative costs attributable to the such services, plus (b) the amount of federal share currently attributable to the state and any certified public expenditures for such services currently attributable to the state and any certified public expenditures for such services and administrative costs; and that such funds shall be designated for the sole purpose of providing mental health services as specified in the Mental Health Master Plan.

The commissioner of Health shall conduct an ongoing evaluation of the mental health services provided under TennCare that includes monthly reports on the number of persons served and the expenditures associated with the provision of such services. The report shall include data on the number of severely and persistently mentally ill persons not covered by TennCare.

16075749 160684

-Page 1 of 1-

Centerstone Community Mental Health Centers, Inc.
CONSUMERS FIRST

Serving Middle Tennessee's Children, Adults and Their Families
With a Broad Range of Integrated Mental Health and Co-Occurrence Services

---

- Establish Middle Tennessee telephone center for intake, triage, appointment scheduling, mobile crisis, *consumer warm line,* information and referral.
- Integrated mobile crisis system for entire region.
- Expanded and improved medical services.
- Expanded and improved respite services and range of housing choices.
- Integrated continuum of outpatient and hospital services.
- Expansion of partial hospitalization, psycho-social, intensive outpatient services and Drop-In Centers *with warm lines connected.*
- Expansion of case management, including "intensive" case management.
- Establish Centerstone Consumer and Family Advocacy Council composed of advocacy leaders who shall provide advice and consultation to management.
- Establish Office of Consumer Affairs, staffed by consumers. Expand Journey of Hope and Bridges training throughout region.
- Establish jail diversion and expand services to the homeless.
- In-home adult services (short-term intensive case management service with a therapeutic and medical component for co-occurrence treatment).
- *Provide education to police and local authorities in regard to needs of mentally ill consumers.*
- Expansion of in-home counseling, case management, preschool, and after-school services to prevent children going into state custody for residential care.
- *Wrap-around services to be provided to include strong case management services for children, parent and community education programs, and parent support groups developed such as Voices vs. Violence.*
- Establish centralized intake, assessment and treatment (EPSDT) of children referred to mental health centers due to demonstration of serious emotional/behavioral problems.

- Provide school-based mental health screening and treatment of students referred because of threats of harm to self or others.
- Establish "Neighborhood Outreach Centers" to improve access of mental health services for residents in areas with little, or no, community support.
- Safety net/regional disaster services coordination.

OBJECTIVES

- Expansion and improvement of quality of services
- Regional integration and improvement in access to services
- Increase in consumer and family satisfaction and their advocacy
- Reduction in state custody and hospitalization for children and adolescents
- Reduction in hospitalization and inappropriate jail placement for adults
- *Reduction in length of time juveniles spend in justice system programs*
- Strengthening of provider and BHO partnership

Italicized topics are incorporated from recommendations made by consumer and family advocacy advisors.

ADMINISTRATIVE OFFICES
COLUMBIA AREA MENTAL HEALTH CENTER
321 WEST SEVENTH ST. — P. O. BOX 1197
COLUMBIA, TENNESSEE 38402-1197

Tel. (615) 381-2335

MEMORANDUM

TO: Members of the Board of Directors
Comprehensive Management Committee

FROM: George Spain GS

DATE: March 24, 1994

RE: Legislative Day, Tennessee Association of Mental Health Centers

---

Your help, and that of the Advisory Boards and Maury County Mental Health Association, resulted in hundreds of letters going to the areas' legislators. When we met with the legislators, we gave them petitions from their constituents. The areas total of 1,052 petition signatures were from the following counties:

Giles	167	Marshall	120
Hickman	25	Maury	471
Lawrence	162	Wayne	41
Lewis	66		

In the letters and petitions, and in our face-to-face meetings with the legislators, there was the strongly expressed concern regarding the inclusion in TennCare of all state and federal funds for mental health services. Now that these funds are not designated for mental health, they can be diminished by using them to pay for other physical services. Our request was that the state and federal funds originally budgeted for mental health be designated in TennCare and used only for mental health services

It was clear that some legislators were not aware that there were no funds specifically ear-marked for mental health. I believe some headway has been made on their realizing what has happened and it has the potential of reducing services to the mentally ill. I believe it will be hard to accomplish our goal of designating funds if the administration strongly opposes it -- but we must try!

Memorandum
March 24, 1994
Page 2

Most of the other Centers had advocates meeting with their legislators. Columbia's board members (Roy & Nita Hamilton, Buck Davis, Steve Saliba, Sandra Thompson, Gloria Quarles, and Mike Greene) were outstanding in their personal support. We owe them much thanks. Hopefully, this state-wide effort will influence the legislature to designate mental health funds.

As we are nowhere near winning this thing, we must, within the next two weeks, continue notifying our legislators of our concern and request their support to an Amendment to the Appropriation Bill. So, here is what I suggest:

1. Keep the letters and phone calls going to your legislators, and get another petition going and mail it.

2. Ask your legislator to request the support of their fellow legislators.

3. Get an article on this in your local newspaper. Tell about the petition and letters. You will find enclosed a copy of my speech which might be used for the article.

4. ****** IMPORTANT ******
   Carefully read the enclosed House Amendment No. 260 which amends the Appropriation Bill so that all state and federal funds budgeted as of December, 1993, are "designated [in TennCare] for the sole purpose of providing mental health services as specified in the Mental Health Master Plan". This Amendment will be sponsored in the House by Rep. John Bragg and in the Senate by Senator Milton Hamilton and John Ford. **IMMEDIATELY** you need to have local people write or call their legislator to support House Amendment No. 260 of the Appropriation Bill.

Clinic Directors, be sure your Advisory Board Members are actively involved in this, also your staff and anyone else supportive of your clinic.

Enclosed are the names of our legislators, the counties they represent, and their addresses and phone numbers.

Also enclosed are the names of legislators serving on the Finance, Ways and Means Committees in the House and Senate. Passage of the Amendment through these committees will be hard. Ask your legislators to personally request their colleagues serving on these committees to support House Amendment No. 260 of the Appropriation Bill.

Thanks for everyone's help. Keep charging!

HOUSE STANDING COMMITTEES

AGRICULTURE 23 LP 741-7001
Bell, Chm.; Givens, Vice-Chm.; Rinks, Sec.; Cross; Ramsey; Walley; Micheal Williams; Windle.

COMMERCE 34 LP 741-1311
Rhinehart, Chm.; Byrd, Vice-Chm.; Jackson, Sec.; Allen; Anderson; Brown; Coffey; Ralph Cole; Ronnie Cole; Draper; Gunnels; Hassell; Haun; McKee; Mires; Moore; Napier; Phelan; Phillips; Pinion; Rigsby; Severance; Shirley; Thompson; Brenda Turner; Venable; L. Mike Williams; Wood.

CONSERVATION AND ENVIRONMENT 22 LP 741-1386
Hillis, Chm.; Cross, Vice-Chm.; Odom, Sec.; Bittle; Brown; Callicott; Crain; Joyce; Kernell; McAfee; Severance; Stulce; Westmoreland.; Micheal Williams; Wix.

CONSUMER AND EMPLOYEE AFFAIRS 37 LP 741-4836
Clark, Chm.; West, Vice-Chm.; Larry Turner, Sec.; Arriola; Joyce; Lewis; Liles; Miller; Shirley; Karen Williams.

EDUCATION 36 LP 741-4811
Davidson, Chm.; Winningham, Vice-Chm.; Ulysses Jones, Sec.; Bell; Boyer; Callicott; Chumney; Davis; Dixon; Draper; Halteman; Knight; McKee; Owenby; Pinion; Ramsey; Ritchie; Stamps; Stulce; Tindell; Whitson.

FINANCE WAYS AND MEANS 33 LP 741-1326
Bragg, Chm.; Kisber, Vice-Chm.; Head, Sec.; Armstrong; Bittle; Byrd; Coffey; Ralph Cole; Collier; Davidson; Garret; Givens; Gunnels; Haun; Hillis; Huskey; Johnson; Rufus Jones; Kent; Love; McDaniel; Moore; Purcell; Rhinehart; Ridgeway; Robinson; Whitson; Winningham; Wix; Wood.

GOVERNMENT OPERATIONS 38 LP 741-4866
Kernell, Chm.; Garrett, Vice-Chm.; Johnson, Sec.; Brooks; Chiles; DeBerry; Haley; McAfee; Owenby.

HEALTH AND HUMAN RESOURCES 17 LP 741-7046
Dixon, Chm.; Pruitt, Vice-Chm.; Armstrong, Sec.; Allen; Arriola; Chiles; DeBerry; Duer; Ferguson; Herron; Jackson; McDaniel; Odom; Brenda Turner; Walley.

JUDICIARY 32 LP 741-1351
Buck, Chm.; Herron, Vice-Chm.; Chumney, Sec.; Clark; Fisher; Hargrove; Purcell; Stamps; Thompson; Karen Williams.

STATE AND LOCAL GOVERNMENT 35 LP 741-4881
Love, Chm.; Rufus Jones, Vice-Chm.; Tindell, Sec.; Fisher; Fowlkes; Halteman; Hargrove; Huskey; Ulysses Jones; Kent; Kisber; Knight; Liles; Meyer; Miller; Phelan; Phillips; Pruitt; Ritchie; Stockburger; West; Westmoreland.

TRANSPORTATION 24 LP 741-1371
Robinson, Chm.; Napier, Vice-Chm.; Fowlkes, Sec.; Anderson; Boyer; Bragg; Brooks; Buck; Ronnie Cole; Collier; Crain; Davis; Duer; Ferguson; Haley; Hassell; Head; Lewis; Meyer; Mires; Ridgeway; Rigsby; Rinks; Stockburger; Larry Turner; Venable; L. Mike Williams; Windle.

CALENDAR AND RULES 20 LP 741-7016
Phillips, Chm.; Brenda Turner, Vice-Chm.; Moore, Sec.

March 14, 1994

Dear

As one of your constituents, I request that you look into problems in TennCare that have the potential for producing major losses in services for mentally ill adults and children with serious emotional disturbances. These problems are:

1. All state and federal funds that were originally intended for mental health services have now been put into TennCare. In 1993 these funds amounted to over $300,000,000. Unless these funds are clearly separated within TennCare, large amounts could be easily diverted from the treatment of mental illness to pay for such physical problems as appendicitis, hernias, ulcers, and gall stones.

   As you know, thousands of state hospital beds no longer exist and, now, most mentally ill children and adults are cared for in the community. If community services are cut due to loss of funds to physical care and there are not enough state hospital beds, where will the mentally ill go? To the streets and to jails. Tennessee is obligated to prevent this! I ask that you support the TennCare Oversight Committee and the Finance Ways & Means Committee looking into this and that you help find a way that assures that the total amount of mental health dollars put into TennCare be used only for mental health services.

2. The Managed Care Organizations do not recognize, nor pay for, community social support services such as housing, supported employment, intensive case management, mobile crisis teams, rehabilitation, etc. These essential services, developed by the state's Master Plan and funded by the Department of Mental Health, will begin to steadily disappear and lead to suffering for the mentally ill. People with severe mental illness cannot be humanely helped in the community with just medicine and counseling. I ask that you support changes in TennCare which set aside community social support funds from hospital and clinical treatment funds.

I will appreciate your seeking information on these issues and sharing what you learn with me. If you find that services for the mentally ill are at risk of being reduced by TennCare, I hope you will take whatever action is necessary to prevent the destruction of a good mental health system which has taken decades to build. And you must let me know what I can do to help you.

With appreciation,

MAR 23 '94 03:09PM TAMHC/CSRI P.2/2

AMENDMENT NO. House #260

FILED
Date
Time
Clerk
Comm. Amdt.

Signature of Sponsor

AMEND Senate Bill No. 2820 **House Bill No.** 2760.

by adding the following new item at the end of Section 10:

Item ___. The commissioner of health shall calculate the total amount of funds for mental health services based on (a) the amount of funds that the bureau of medicaid and the department of mental health and mental retardation budgeted, as of December 31, 1993, for (1) those mental health services that are now covered by TennCare benefits and (2) administrative costs attributable to the such services, plus (b) the amount of federal share currently attributable to the state and any certified public expenditures for such services currently attributable to the state and any certified public expenditures for such services and administrative costs; and that such funds shall be designated for the sole purpose of providing mental health services as specified in the Mental Health Master Plan.

The commissioner of Health shall conduct an ongoing evaluation of the mental health services provided under TennCare that includes monthly reports on the number of persons served and the expenditures associated with the provision of such services. The report shall include data on the number of severely and persistently mentally ill persons not covered by TennCare.

16075749 160684

-Page 1 of 1-

SENATE STANDING COMMITTEES

COMMERCE LABOR AND AGRICULTURE 309 WMB 741-7061
Koella, Chm.; Cooper, Vice-Chm.; Wallace, Sec.; Albright; Crutchfield; Elsea; O'Brien; Patten; Rochelle.

EDUCATION 2 LP 741-3038
Albright, Chm.; Womack, Vice-Chm.; Burks, Sec.; Atchley; Elsea; Kyle; Leatherwood; O'Brien; Springer.

ENERGY AND NATURAL RESOURCES 307 WMB 741-3536
Greer, Chm.; Kyle, Vice-Chm.; Leatherwood, Sec.; Burks; Crowe; Hamilton; McNally, Rice; Wallace.

FINANCE, WAYS AND MEANS 11 LP 741-7881
Henry, Chm.; McNally, Vice-Chm.; Rochelle, Sec.; Atchley; Crutchfield; Ford; Hamilton; Patten; Womack.

GENERAL WELFARE, HEALTH AND HUMAN RESOURCES 7 LP 741-7936
Ford, Chm.; Holcomb, Vice-Chm.; Patten, Sec.; Cooper; Crutchfield; Hamilton; Henry; Koella; Person.

GOVERNMENT OPERATIONS 5 LP 741-3642
Haynes, Chm.; Rice, Vice-Chm.; Springer, Sec.; Davis; Elsea; Harper; Holcomb; Leatherwood; McKnight; Wallace; Wright.

JUDICIARY 308 WMB 741-7821
Person, Chm.; Jordan, Vice-Chm.; Crowe, Sec.; Cohen; Gilbert; Harper; Haynes; Holcomb; O'Brien.

STATE AND LOCAL GOVERNMENT 8 LP 741-4108
Cohen, Chm.; Harper, Vice-Chm.; Gilbert, Sec.; Greer; Haynes; Koella; McKnight; Rochelle; Womack.

TRANSPORTATION 321 WMB 741-7971
Davis, Chm.; McKnight, Vice-Chm.; Wright, Sec.; Cooper; Crowe; Gilbert; Jordan; Rice; Springer.

CALENDAR 13 LP 741-3145
Hamilton, Chm.; Atchley; Crutchfield.

10

PERSONAL INDEX OF THE HOUSE

15
15/0

98th General Assembly
Speaker of the House

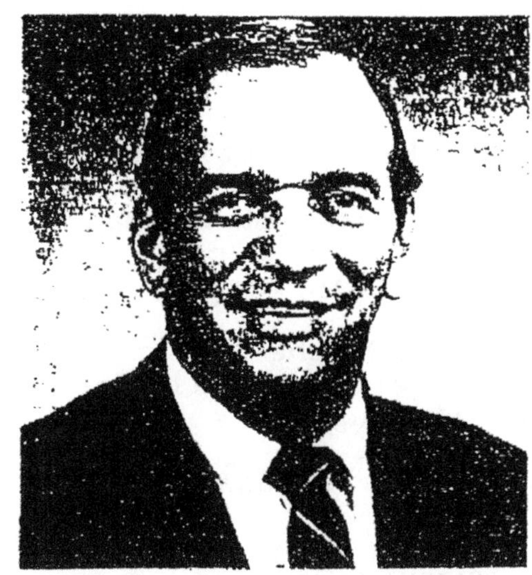

(99) **REP. JIMMY NAIFEH (D)—(81)**
Leg. Office: 19 LP
Nashville 37243-0181 615-741-3774
Office: P.O. Box 97
Covington 38019 901-476-9593
Res.: P.O. Box 97
Covington 38019 901-476-9591
Occupation: Businessman

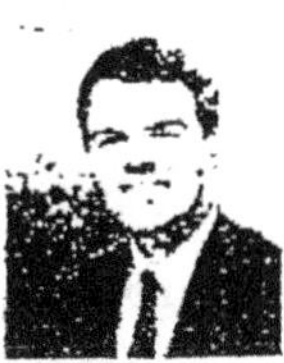

(51) **REP. CHARLES E. ALLEN, JR. (R)—(6)**
Spouse: Barbara Leg. Office: 212 WMB
Nashville 37243-0106 615-741-1897
Office: 3300 Browns Mill Road
Johnson City 37604 615-282-9100
Res.: 3300 Browns Mill Road
Johnson City 37604 615-282-3735
Occupation: Businessman and CPA

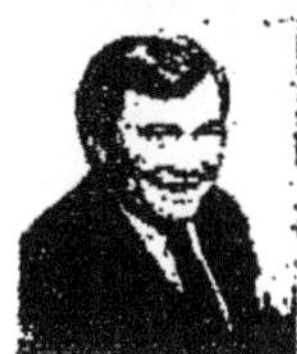

(63) **REP. W. TOWNSEND ANDERSON (R)—(20)**
Spouse: Jeannie Leg. Office: 206 WMB
Nashville 37243-0120 615-741-0751
Res.: 1116 N. Heritage Drive
Maryville 37801 615-984-5542
Occupation: Businessman

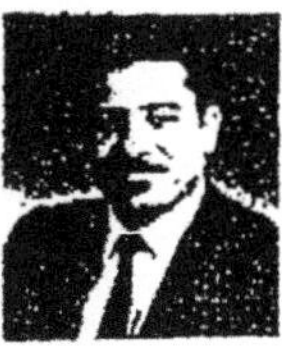

(29) **REP. JOSEPH ARMSTRONG (D)—(15)**
Leg. Office: 17 LP
Nashville 37243-0115 615-741-0768
Office: 4520 Ashville Hwy.
Knoxville 37914 615-522-9268
Res.: 2624 Selma Avenue
Knoxville 37914 615-523-6374
Occupation: District Manager Insurance

◯ Indicate seat number 11 ( ) Indicate district

PETITION TO THE TENNESSEE LEGISLATURE

WHEREAS, Tennessee's state and federal funds are no longer specifically designated within the state budget to provide services for mentally ill adults and seriously emotionally disturbed children,

AND WHEREAS these funds are now made part of TennCare they can be readily diverted to pay for physical health care,

AND WHEREAS TennCare's Managed Care Organizations do not pay for community support services, such as housing, supported employment, intensive case management, mobile crisis teams, drop in centers, rehabilitation, etc., which are essential to help people with mental illness remain in the community,

AND WHEREAS the reduction in funds formerly available for mental health services will reduce hospital and clinic treatment and community support services,

AND WHEREAS thousands of beds have been eliminated from the state hospitals,

AND WHEREAS the reduction in state hospital beds and community services will produce suffering for the mentally ill and increase their jail admissions and homelessness,

We now therefore, as residents of Tennessee, request that the Legialature assure that the full amount of state and federal funds originally intended for mental health services, be set aside in TennCare and be used only for helping mentally ill adults and seriously emotionally disturbed children,

And that an appropriate portion of these funds be specifically designated to pay for community, social support services which help the mentally ill achieve independence and live humanely in their communities.

SJR61 LEGISLATIVE COMMITTEE

TESTIMONY PRESENTED OCTOBER 7, 1997

BY GEORGE SPAIN

Senator Henry, Members of the Mental Health Study Committee

My name is George Spain. I am a native Tennessean and have worked for forty years in mental health in middle Tennessee, first at the old Davidson County Psychiatric Hospital, then Central State Hospital (now MTMHI), then for eight years in child psychiatry at Vanderbilt, and for the past thirty years at the Columbia Area community Mental Health Center. Since this past February, I have served as the CEO of Pinnacle Health, a non profit company which serves Harriett Cohn, Highland Rim and Columbia Area Mental Health Centers.

I began working in mental health only five years after Governor Frank Clement established the Department of Mental Health in 1953. It was one of the first such departments in the nation. Historically, the state hospitals had been administered by the same department that oversaw prisons and reformatories. Clement realized that the appalling conditions that he had observed in the hospitals in 1952 would likely not change unless there was leadership from a separate cabinet level department. He was also influenced by a family tragedy - an uncle who was living in a state hospital as the result of a gunshot injury to his brain.

I want to talk with you about human tragedy and disaster and my fear that community mental health centers cannot respond in the future as they have in the past. Until now, Tennesseans could be assured that across this state there was a safety net of services available at the centers. The centers, through their state contracts and grant funding, were required to provide disaster response services. Let me list a few, several of which I was personally involved with. In each one a mental health center provided extensive services to individuals and their families.

SUMMER, 1977 Waverly train wreck and fire, 8 die (including Chief of Police), Mental Health Clinic destroyed. Harriett Cohn Mental Health Center

Maury County Jail fire, 42 die, many of whom were visitors. Columbia Area Mental Health Center

DECEMBER, 1986 Lawrence County boarding home fire, 7 die Columbia Area Mental Health Center

FEBRUARY, 1987 Lawrence County boarding home fire, 27 mentally ill patients homeless put up in motel. Columbia Area Center was recognized by Governor McWherter and House of Representatives.

*AUGUST 24, 1992 Miami, Hurricane Andrew, 52 die. Four Tennessee Mental Health Centers sent three teams to help victims. Harriett Cohn, Vanderbilt, Luton, and Columbia Area.

<u>JANUARY, 1994</u> Clarksville, Taco Bell robbery, 4 killed. Harriett Cohn Mental Health Center

<u>APRIL, 1994</u> Nashville, John Trotwood Moore, 11 year old boy killed by fellow student. Dede Wallace Center

<u>MAY, 1995</u> Lawrence County tornado kills 3. Columbia Area Mental Health Center

<u>NOVEMBER, 1995</u> Giles County, Richland School. A student and teacher are shot to death by a student. Columbia Area Center recognized by Commissioner of Department of Mental Health and Department of Education.

<u>FEBRUARY, 1996</u> Donelson. Navy plane crash kills 5. Luton Mental Health Center

Then, there are the innumerable individual and family tragedies and disasters that receive little to no news coverage, such as a friend of mine and my wife who one afternoon went to her garden and shot herself in the head. Later on in the day she was found by her husband who was left with two young sons.

Tennessee's CMHCs have always been there to respond to these human tragedies and disasters. But will this be so in the future? This need and service is not addressed in TennCare nor Tenn Care Partners. At present, there is no expectation nor funding that assures that such services will be available across the state. It is a significant oversight which I hope this committee will address in its recommendations.

JUDGE JOHN STANTON
FUNERAL SERVICES
DECEMBER 28, 1997
EULOGY BY GEORGE SPAIN

Polly, thank you for the honor you have given me to speak here today.

To you, your children, your grandchildren - it was an honor to have been the friend of Judge John Stanton - a wise and good man of great integrity, who believed strongly in individual responsibility - yet believed equally in helping others who had problems making their way in life.

In 1831, 147 Maury Countians were the first people in Tennessee to petition the Legislature for the mentally ill, the lunatics as they were then called. They saw the appalling conditions of these ill people in this county and influenced the building of the first hospital in Tennessee for their care.

One hundred and thirty-seven years later, in 1968, I came with three others to the Maury County Mental Health Clinic to work with the mentally ill and families with problems. Judge Stanton played a major part in our coming.

He was one of the first people I met. He was one of my bosses - as as a member of the clinics board of directors. Soon I began working with him in his position as juvenile judge.

In those days, the county judge held great power as both county executive, juvenile judge, and as the one who had to sign papers for the commitment of a mentally ill person to the state hospital. Not only did I hold Judge Stanton in awe, but I felt somewhat intimidated by him. I remember that I sure did not want him ever to get angry at me.

I occasionally sat in juvenile court at his request to see if the clinic could help any of the teenagers and children who came before him or their families. I remember a sullen, ill mannered, lying teenager who appeared before him, Judge Stanton, - "Young man, do not purger yourself to this court...if everytime someone committed purgery, a brick fell off this court house, we would now be sitting in a pile of rubble. So, do not purger yourself". He later referred him to the clinic.

It soon became evident to me that Judge Stanton was different than most juvenile judges of that time. Rather than quickly dismissing children by sending them off to Jordonia or the Tennessee Preparatory School, he sought ways to help them and their families in the community if he felt there was any hope. He developed one of the first systems that made major use of evaluations of children and of family counseling.

Then in 1970, he was chosen by the governor and President as one of 50 Tennesseeans to attend the first White House Conference on Children. From that experience, in April, 1971 at Maury County Park Kiwanis Shelter (brown bag lunch) he invited all the major community agencies. Agencies represented were: Schools, Welfare Department, Employment Security, Vocational Rehabilitation, Mental Health, Ministerial Association, Public Health, and Juvenile Probation. At this meeting we formed the Maury County Council on Families to help in the community families with the most difficult

problems. **This was a new idea in Tennessee.**
The councils success and fame resulted in many other Tennessee counties requesting information and coming to learn in order to set up their own council. This brought Judge Stanton acclaim with the Tennessee Department of Mental Health and Mental Retardation and the Tennessee Juvenile Judges Association.

At the same time, Judge Stanton had become one of the areas leaders in supporting the spread of mental health services to other rural counties. He helped found the Columbia Area Mental Health Center in 1972, which received federal funds to serve eight counties. Recently the Columbia Center provided the leadership which connected 4 centers together. The new company, Centerstone Community Mental Health Centers, Inc., now serves 23 counties of middle Tennessee, with 800 employees and over 30,000 clients in one year. Judge Stanton helped lay the foundation for this largest mental health center in Tennessee.

Recognized for his leadership in mental health, he was appointed many years ago to the Board of Trustees for the Tennessee Department of Mental Health-Mental Retardation where he worked with several commissioners and governors, all who held him in high esteem.

A couple of personal notes - we both loved to read and shared books and book reviews - he read good books almost to the end, (Davis

Kidd - Biography on **Whittaker Chambers).**

And once in a rough time in my life, when I was down, and disheartened, I went to him to pour out my problems and my self blame and he listened, as my friend - and did not turn away, nor did he lose faith in me thereafter. I will never forget him for this one thing alone.

Judge John Stanton rose above most of us in facing head on some of the most severe problems confronting society - adult crime, juvenile delinquency and mental illness. In his time, on this earth, he gave his time, energy and wisdom to try to make things better for us, with particular attention for those people most difficult to help.

So here, for this moment, let us seize hold of his memory, to inspire us all to be a little stronger, and a little better in helping others and in doing so, we help ourselves.

It is fitting to close with a quote from a book, David McCullough's - **Truman**

Of Truman's life, McCullough summarizes:

> "He held to the old guidelines: work hard, do your best, speak the truth, assume no airs, trust in God, have no fear".

And paraphrasing now from Truman, I say -

> "I'm not sure Judge Stanton was right about everything. But remembering him reminds me what a man ought to be like. Its character, just character. Now, he stands like a rock in my memory".

State should boost mental health care: principal

By Steven Susens
BANNER POLITICAL WRITER

It's been two years since Jamie Rouse walked into Richland School with a loaded semiautomatic rifle and killed two teachers and another student.

But for a second-grade student who watched as his teacher was shot, the nightmares still linger, says Ron Shirey, an assistant principal at the school and one of Rouse's intended targets in the November 1995 shooting.

The school suffers yet from the shooting, and the mental health services that were crucial in the immediate aftermath of the tragedy are still needed, Shirey testified Wednesday before a special joint committee of the General Assembly looking at the accessibility of mental health programs in the state and the current funding systems for programs providing mental health to the "working poor."

"School guidance (counselors) are generally not prepared to handle this type of trauma," Shirey said. "The limited number of school psychologists that we may have in a rural area, such as ours, would be overwhelmed with the amount of people seeking help and reassurance at the time.

"We would have made out, I'm sure. But, not as quickly or as carefully as was handled through the mental health professionals."

Immediate help

As soon as the shootings occurred, mental health officials in Giles County began setting up counseling sessions at the school and talking with students, family members and faculty about the tragic events and what they were experiencing.

It was the immediate and coordinated help of Barabara Conrad, Giles County Mental health director, that helped heal some of the wounds in the incident, but the lingering effects can still be felt, Shirey said.

Although the mental health services after the Lynnville shootings were available, some mental health experts say that availability is dwindling under a managed care system.

"A few years ago, it would be guaranteed that we could provide those services, especially in a disaster," said George Spain, chief executive officer for Centerstone Community Mental Health Centers. "But under a managed care system, there are just no resources for those kinds of services."

Spain has been advocating for more state resources in providing mental health services for the working poor. He testified that the opportunities for the poor who need mental health services are becoming harder to find.

"When the state turned over their health care to a managed care system, they did not address disaster relief, such as what happened in Giles County," Spain said. "So, we've been trying to bring that back to the attention of the state to get the resources we need."

Chris Wyre, executive director of the Guidance Center Mental Health Clinics, said the mental health professionals in the state are always being called out for disaster help, such as devastation from tornadoes, shootings and au-

Please see **MENTAL**, page A18

Thursday, January 8, 1998

Mental

Continued from page A17

tomobile accidents, but that the managed care structure does not offer adequate help in dealing with the number of people affected by these type of events.

"It's like a juggling act, but we used to be able to juggle better than what we can do now," Wyre said.

Mental health services for disasters is only one program hampered by the current system, officials said.

Debbie Hillin, president of the Tennessee Alcohol and Drug Association, testified that the majority of treatment options being made available for those addicted to controlled substances are on an outpatient basis, which is not adequately addressing the problems.

A licensed drug and alcohol therapist herself, Hillin said many of the clients she helps need more than 12 to 14 therapy sessions on an outpatient basis, which does not help the more dependent addicts to a full recovery.

"I'm not going to tell you that a 28-day inpatient recovery program is the answer for everyone, but the longer I can keep that in a combination of care treatments, the greater the chances to get them on a more substantial recovery,"

John Ferguson, Commissioner of Finance and Administration, says although a number of programs were phased out when the state adopted the managed care system, quality care is still the primary goal.

"To some, it may look like we have cut these programs because we are trying to cover more people on an outpatient basis, but the truth is that the programs are still there and we provide the services we always had," Ferguson said.

Steven Susens may be reached at 255-6287 or by e-mail: ssusens@NashvilleBanner.com

THE TENNESSEAN
PERSPECTIVE
SUNDAY, FEBRUARY 1, 1998

Up in arms over state handling of mental health, retardation

By ELLEN DAHNKE
Staff Writer

Forty-five years after Gov. Frank Clement gave the mentally ill a voice in state government, advocates are wondering where it went.

Mental health and retardation services in Tennessee are under siege. Gov. Don Sundquist's plan to merge the Department of Mental Health and Mental Retardation with the Department of Health might have been expected to engender opposition from advocates who saw the Cabinet-level position as a voice at the table of public policy.

But the uproar over the other partnership in mental health services announced by the governor — TennCare Partners — has all but overwhelmed any calm discussion about the merger.

The consensus seems to be that the state took on more than could reasonably be expected to work in a short amount of time.

"I think the state is trying to do too much at one time," said George Spain, chief executive officer of Centerstone Community Mental Health Centers Inc. (formerly Pinnacle and Dede Wallace) and a life-long mental health advocate. "It's like whitewater rafting on the highest rated stream — you let one raft go through at a time, or you risk disaster."

Spain, a student of the history of mental health policy in Tennessee, acknowledges that advocates have traditionally had to fight for attention as well as money — even after Clement's landmark establishment of the department.

For Clement, the issue was personal. An uncle had been placed in an institution after a gunshot wound to the head. Tennessee's institutionalized weren't far removed from the Hollywood image in *The Snake Pit*, Spain noted.

There was no treatment. People with any kind of mental disease or disability were put out of sight and out of the public mind. Indeed, there was no department at all: The facilities were in the same department as prisons and other state institutions.

Dr. Frank Luton of Vanderbilt University was among the first to call for a separate state division dedicated to mental health and headed by a psychiatrist in 1938. But it wasn't until Clement cam-

Turn to PAGE 2D Column 1

Up in arms over state handling of

FROM PAGE 1D

paigned and won the 1952 election for governor that any steps were taken.

Much of Clement's legacy has been tattered over the years, but even his opponents credit his establishment of the Department of Mental Health as a major and lasting achievement for him and the state he represented. It was one of the first separate departments in the United States.

"There was a great deal of pride that Tennessee was a leader in mental health at that time," Spain said.

It also coincided with an important development in treating mental illness — a generation of drugs aimed at controlling some of the symptoms of mental disorders. For example, thorazine was used to help those diagnosed with schizophrenia.

By the time Dr. Nat Winston, who would later become mental health commissioner, opened the trailblazing Moccasin Bend hospital in Chattanooga in the 1960s, the contrast with treatment just a decade before was immense, he recalled.

"It was a showplace," Winston said. And what psychiatric professionals were able to show to the state was a place where patients could have mirrors or use a knife and fork without fear that they would harm themselves. Clement rewarded Winston by later appointing him commissioner.

The use of drugs and therapy also meant the state could begin to empty the hospitals it had built to house the mentally ill. At its peak in the 1960s, Tennessee had more than 8,000 patients in its hospitals for the mentally ill. Today, it has about one-tenth that many.

But as those patients left the hospitals, the state failed to provide for all the services they needed out in the community, critics said, and that, in part, caused the great migration of mentally ill to the streets.

Part of the problem in sustaining interest in the legislature over the years may rest in the divided constituency that mental health and mental retardation advocates represent. The settlement of the lawsuit over Arlington Developmental Center shifted more of the attention in recent years to mental retardation and disabilities advocates. Even advocates are divided among themselves about whether those formerly in the centers can be treated in community-based care.

But it was that settlement that led the governor to propose the changes in the system now under fire. Carol Westlake, executive director of the Tennessee Coalition for the Disabled, an organization of some 56 different advocacy groups, has been one of the more vocal opponents in discussions about both the merger of the department and TennCare Partners. She acknowledges that there are often conflicting interests with advocates for the mentally ill.

"But one of the real concerns on both sides is that we think it's important that there be a person at the Cabinet-level who goes to bed at night and wakes up in the morning thinking about mental health, men-

f mental health and retardation

tal retardation and developmental disabilities."

If the state wasn't thinking about those problems before, the administration has hardly been able to escape it for the last several months. The final stages of the merger of the two departments await the action of the legislature. Senate hearings have already begun on that.

But the issue has been overshadowed by the legislature's TennCare Oversight Committee, chaired by Sen. Roy Herron, D-Dresden. Since last year, the committee has heard professionals, advocates and even sheriffs complain that TennCare Partners, the $350 million offshoot of TennCare for mental health services, has been a failure.

Sheriffs, including Sheriff Gayle Ray of Nashville, complained that the mentally ill are filling up their jails. Community health centers made desperate pleas to lawmakers for emergency payments because the Partners program was underfunded. Advocates have provided their own horror stories of people being neglected or turned away for treatment.

As the reviews the performance of the two behavioral health organizations providing TennCare Partners—Premier Health Services Inc. and Tennessee Behavioral Health—serious problems have shown up. Even more embarrassing, the reports were done in September and October and not made public by the state until the Memphis *Commercial Appeal* asked about them last week. At the same time, the reports were forwarded to the Health Care Financing Administration which is expected to release its own review of the situation soon.

But Commissioner of Health Nancy Menke, who's been under constant fire from the legislature almost since she was first appointed last year, vigorously defends the state's actions.

"We've been too busy solving problems to publish reports," Menke insisted. Measures have already been implemented, she said, to provide better monitoring and improved services. Among the efforts are "aggressive measures" to ensure appropriate discharge and case management procedures by the BHOs, shortcomings cited by the report.

Herron disputes Menke's claims.

"I have not heard any testimony this summer or this fall that indicates the quality of care for mental illness or alcohol and substance abuse is anywhere remotely like it needs to be," Herron said. "We're not just losing the war on drugs, we're surrendering."

Gordon Bonnyman, a lawyer who's lobbied in the past on a variety of health-care issues for the poor, takes issue with the timing of the merger while "the state is in flames." The state's acting on the developmental centers at the point of a judge's and the federal government's gun. And, the problems of TennCare Partners has the state putting out one fire after another. He said, however, that he thinks true managed care should be given a chance to work. ■

JOINT STUDY COMMITTEE ON MENTAL HEALTH DELIVERY SYSTEMS (SJR 161)

TESTIMONY PRESENTED JANUARY 7, 1998

BY GEORGE SPAIN, CEO

CENTERSTONE COMMUNITY MENTAL HEALTH CENTERS, INC.

Senator Henry, members of the committee, thank you for the opportunity to again address you as you continue to study the mental health system in preparation for recommendations to the 1998 General Assembly. In the handout is a copy of a December 29, 1997 Nashville Banner article, by Mr. Bill Synder, entitled, Mentally ill inmates fill more jail cells. I believe it is an excellent and accurate article, one that likely applies to the greater part of Tennessee. If, indeed, it is accurate, that there is a major increase of mentally ill people being kept in our jails because of "declining funding for mental health services", then something is going seriously awry in Tennessee - for these are the headlines of days long gone by. This was a major concern expressed by Dorothea Dix 150 years ago in her memorial to the Tennessee General Assembly for the improvement of care to the mentally ill. And this was a major concern of Frank Clement forty-five years ago when he established the Department of Mental Health. Yes, there are some things gone terribly awry in our mental health system and we, who are advocates for the mentally ill, seriously emotionally disturbed and people suffering from a substance abuse illness look forward to your recommendations for improvements.

You have asked me to respond to two questions and then to describe the impact resulting from the affiliation of four middle Tennessee

Page two

mental health centers to form Centerstone Community Mental Health Centers, Inc.

First your two questions:

1. "Should the state of Tennessee fund a general behavioral health care system (i.e., a safety net) for the uninsured and working poor who are not TennCare eligible and who are unable to afford the full cost of such services?"

   Yes. Services to these people have been either drastically reduced or eliminated, potentially resulting in increased suicide, increased drug or alcohol abuse, extreme neglect or abuse of their families. And, as we see with increasing frequency: violence and murder. These are not people sometimes referred to as the "worried well" but are those who have experienced major traumas in their lives.

   Funding recommendation: As with several states (Kentucky, North Carolina, Colorado, Arizona) some state funding should be established for services for these people. Consideration should also be given to local matching funds and clients paying a portion on a sliding scale.

2. "Should the state of Tennessee fund a community based response system to provide disaster related mental health counseling and support services?"

   Yes. Dr. Robert Vero and I presented testimony to this serious need on October 7, 1997. As the community mental health centers have the only statewide network and, until recently, had this responsibility as part of our state

Page three

contracts, disaster counseling and support services should be provided by the centers.

Funding recommendation: State grant funding should assure statewide availability, equity in distribution, and integration with state disaster plans and resources.

Now, let me provide you information on Centerstone and its impact on staff and services;

1. What is Centerstone Community Mental Health Centers, Inc.?

- Not for profit corporation. 501 (c) (3)
- It is a parent company (legally a "sole member") that provides administrative support and direction to four community mental health centers who retain their local name and identity:
  - Columbia Area Mental Health Center
  - Dede Wallace Center
  - Harriett Cohn Mental Health Center
  - Highland Rim Mental Health Center
- Centerstone is the largest community mental health center provider in Tennessee:
  - Provides services in 23 counties
  - 25 percent of entire TennCare population lives in its service area
  - 800 employees
  - $32,000,000 budget for Tennessee based services
- Operated by a single board of directors, twenty-two members selected from the four Center boards.
- Shares financial risk and has a single management team for its

Page four

operations.

- Has authority to contract for its member centers.
- Incentives and polices are aligned to promote coordination.
- Has a Board of Trustees composed of twenty county executives and one Development Board (soon four) for funding raising and advocacy.
- See brochure with the handout for additional information.

2. Why was Centerstone created?
   - First and foremost, to enable the four centers to improve client care. Secondly, to enhance our mission as non profit community mental health centers governed by a board of Tennessee volunteer directors. We could not accept other options: becoming part of a hospital as occurred with three other centers or failure such as Spectra in Memphis.
   - To improve overall efficiency and effectiveness. We have already saved several hundred thousand dollars in premiums, supply purchasing and computer development.
   - To combine management for enhancement in the quality of services and contracting power.
   - To increase size and financial resources in preparation for considering direct contracting with the state thereby removing one of the layers of existing administrative cost.

Page five

- To strengthen our voice and influence as advocate for those who are mentally ill, severally emotionally disturbed, or abusers of alcohol and drugs.

3. How does Centerstone impact staff delivery and service efficiency?

There is a larger pool of talent and resources to draw from:

- Dede Wallace is strong in children services while the other centers are strong in adult services.
- Dede Wallace has one of the best computer systems in Tennessee.
- Columbia, Harriett, and Highland provide large population and geography for service expansion.
- Most experienced staff have been selected from the four centers for management positions.
- Quality and continuity enhanced by single standards and policies. Best practices cross-pollinate throughout the system.
- Reduction in program directors from four to one
- Frees staff to expand into new services i.e., geriatrics, commercial, etc.
- With prior boundaries eliminated, staff can be shifted to where need arises.
- Specialized programs of one center now available to all four centers.

Last, you asked me to address "other issues affected by the advent of managed care:

NASHVILLE BANNER 12/29/97

Mentally ill inmates fill more jail cells

By Bill Snyder
BANNER SENIOR MEDICAL WRITER

The number of mentally ill people taken to jail in Nashville appears to be rising, despite the efforts to tackle the problem.

"It's not fair," says Metro Sheriff Gayle Ray. "Jail is not the place for a mentally ill person to get better."

Last February, for example, 121 inmates in the Criminal Justice Center, more than 15 percent of the total jail population, were receiving psychiatric drugs for treatment of mental illnesses, according to the Metro Sheriff's Department.

> "It's not fair. Jail is not the place for a mentally ill person to get better.
>
> Gayle Ray
> Metro sheriff

Earlier this month, that number had grown to 190 inmates, about 30 percent of the jail population.

Last February, 23 inmates were on close observation because they had previously threatened or attempted suicide. Earlier this month, that figure had risen to 29 inmates.

Experts say the downsizing of psychiatric hospitals, and declining funding for mental health services contribute to the problem, not only here but throughout the country.

In addition, some psychiatrists claim that TennCare Partners, the state program that provides mental health and substance abuse benefits for many low-income Tennesseans, has made matters worse by not adequately funding services, and by setting up incentives to drop difficult and costly patients into jail.

Most people with mental illness do not commit crimes. But those who do often are difficult and costly to treat, says Jeff Blum, a program specialist with the Metro Public Defender's Office.

Inmates

Continued from page A1

For example, the Metro jail inmates have been charged with crimes ranging from indecent exposure to murder, and half of them had substance abuse problems in addition to mental illness.

As a result, many insurance programs — public as well as private — probably are "just as happy to have them in jail," Blum asserts. Instead of the insurer paying for treatment, Metro government — which is responsible for providing health services to inmates — must now pick up the tab, he says.

But this is not just a problem with insurance or TennCare, asserts Dr. Roy Sanders, medical director of the Mental Health Co-operative, which provides case management to mentally ill people in Nashville.

Nearly all of the agency's clients who end up in jail are there because of drug-related issues, "rarely because of psychosis alone," Sanders says.

"Until we address the crack problem in the housing projects, we are never going to get at the core of the problem," he says.

Mentally ill people who don't have family or financial support often wind up in public housing, Sanders says, where there is "a drug and alcohol epidemic."

Because they are the most vulnerable to becoming involved in drug-related activities, "they're the ones who wind up in jail," he says.

In addition to attacking the substance abuse problem in public housing, Sanders envisions a three-pronged approach to reducing the number of mentally ill people in jail:

- Establish a place for the police to take people to be evaluated for mental illness, instead of sending them to jail.
- Develop all levels of housing for people with mental illness.
- Train police, the jail and courts to deal more effectively with people with mental illness.

Sanders has his own critics, however.

A video on TennCare Partners produced this fall for the Tennessee Psychiatric Association claims that the Mental Health Co-op contributes to the problem by housing mentally ill people in local motels without proper supervision, and by discouraging patients — against the advice of their psychiatrist — from admitting themselves to psychiatric hospitals.

Psychiatrists interviewed on the video speculated that the goal is to save TennCare money, rather than provide proper treatment for patients.

Sanders admits that mentally ill people often are placed in a "respite program" in local motels as an alternative to hospitalization. But he argues that these people are adequately supervised.

He admits that his agency discourages hospitalization but not to save money for TennCare. "Research shows the consumers and patients do better when they are in a friendlier and (less restrictive) environment," he says.

Sanders points out that psychiatrists make more money when they admit patients to the hospital.

There have been some failures with respite, but, says Sanders, "There have been a lot more successes."

Lack of services

Law enforcement officials remain frustrated, however, by the difficulty in obtaining services for mentally ill inmates — or even obtaining psychiatric evaluations for them in the first place.

"Unless they're literally playing out in traffic on the interstate," it's "almost impossible" to get a mental health evaluation approved for an indigent person, says General Sessions Judge Penny Harrington, who hears petitions for involuntary psychiatric commitment.

Harrington says she does not want to go back to the 1950s, when it was too easy to get people admitted involuntarily to psychiatric hospitals. But "now we've got people who are in clear need of assistance ... and we're depriving them of proper treatment," she says.

Another problem is lack of services once they leave jail, Harrington says.

"We don't want them on the streets for humanitarian reasons, and because many of them are unable to care for themselves," she says. "But there is no place for them to live. It's scary."

"If the Co-op is able to get there (to the scene of a disturbance), then they can work with the police and hopefully get this person calmed down, maybe get their medication, possibly even take them to a motel or somewhere for a few days to get them stabilized," Sheriff Ray says.

"But as I understand it, the Co-op is so understaffed that they are almost never able to get there in a tim.ely manner. So the police have pretty much given up on that deal, and they just go ahead and run the person to jail."

Sanders admits the TennCare funding crunch has made his agency's job increasingly difficult. But he adds that the police and mental health providers need to work more closely together to get the mentally ill where they need to go.

New programs

Local authorities are developing new programs to cope with the press of mentally ill inmates. Among them is a jail treatment program for inmates who have both mental illness and substance-abuse problems.

In addition, Park Center, a nonprofit organization in Nashville that provides services to people with mental illness, will open a new, 20-bed residential program for the homeless mentally ill early next year.

The program will work with the Sheriff's Department to help "stabilize" people who have not been charged with violent offenses.

"This is something that we have not had before," says Bill Hampton, director of programs for the Sheriff's Department. "When a person is released from our institution, sometimes they're back the next day or the day they're released."

The Park Center program "is a transitional place for the mentally ill to go once they're released ... to help them get a place to stay, possibly a job, get on their medication, get all the resources in place — and to follow those people and hope that they will become successful and not return," Hampton says.

Ray says she worries that the jail will become — more and more — a treatment facility.

"It seems like the more services you offer, the more the court system and everyone else will start to see it as being appropriate to leave people or put people in jail for these problems," she says.

That's not good for the patient.

Mentally ill inmates "tend to deteriorate more when they're in jail," Hampton says. "I call it a cycle of self-destruction."

Sanders agrees. Unless this problem is solved, "It's going to bring us all down," he says.

"There won't be a comprehensive system. Money will run out and people won't get the care they need."

Bill Snyder may be reached at 259-8226 or by e-mail: bsnyder@NashvilleBanner.com

Senate Government Operations Committee

Testimony Regarding Merger of Tennessee Department of Mental Health and Mental Retardation into Tennessee Department of Health (SB1925/HB1827)

By George Spain, CEO

Centerstone Community Mental Health Centers, Inc.

February 18, 1998

Senator Springer, members of the Committee, thank you for this opportunity to speak on the proposed merger of the Department of Mental Health and Mental Retardation into the Department of Health.

I have worked for forty years in mental health in Tennessee, almost from the time of Governor Frank Clement's creation of the Department of Mental Health in 1953. Senator O'Brien helped me get my first job. I have seen much change; many improvements. In the past eighteen months, I have participated in the bringing together of four mental health centers to create Centerstone Community Mental Health Centers, Inc., the largest provider of mental health services in Tennessee.

There is a good reason for merging the Departments. It can help bring mental health services and treatment into the mainstream of health care. Schizophrenia and bi-polar disorders are brain illnesses. They are chronic illnesses like Parkinson's disease or diabetes. While there is still no cure for them, there is control of the symptoms and the possibility of living a satisfying and productive life. The more we see mental illness as illness the more it helps diminish prejudice and stigma. New medicines and social services are greatly improving the lives of our family members, friends and neighbors who have mental illness. The merger of the Departments should help in the coordination and development of medical services for the mentally ill. If the merger occurs the Department of Health must also assure that special support and rehabilitation services are continued, such as: case management, supported employment, psychosocial rehabilitation and housing.

With all of this said, the timing and rush on this is highly questionable. You have heard little evidence that shows comprehensive, broad based planning having been done for this merger and yet we are rushing toward its happening. As Senator O'Brien recalled, the decision to create the Department of Mental Health in 1953 was a seriously considered decision – should not the decision to abolish the Department be given equally serious thought?

You know Tennessee has some serious, very serious problems with the Partner's program, which must be our priority whether or not this merger occurs. You have heard many speak against the merger, and Senator Williams rightly asks if there is displeasure with what exists and opposition to the merger, then what is to be done?

Rather than add to the drum roll you have heard of problems and criticisms, I would like to offer some specific recommendations. They will be related to mental health and alcohol and drug services as I am neither experienced nor knowledgeable in mental retardation nor developmental disabilities. My recommendations are:

1. Delay for one year the statutory obliteration of the Department of Mental Health and Mental Retardation. During this year give the Department of Health, which already has the staff and money transferred to it, the chance to prove itself. See if it can show substantial evidence that it can provide successful leadership. If it cannot, then return the staff and money to TDMH-MR and have the Governor appoint a full-time commissioner.

2. A major piece of evidence for judging failure or success will be the Department's ability to clean up the mess that exists with the Partner's program. You should expect substantial improvement.

3. The Department of Health will soon receive a brief report with general recommendations from a Master Plan Task Force. Developing a new, updated Master Plan should be a major priority. Commissioner Menke should contract with Mary Rolando, former assistant commissioner of Mental Health who led the development of the original Master Plan to develop a new, comprehensive Master Plan. The Statewide Planning Council of DMH-MR should be involved in the development of the Plan.

4. In like manner, a detailed alcohol and drug plan, which is developed with broad representative assistance, is needed. There is a strong belief that A&D planning and services have diminished since the transfer from DMH-MR to the Department of Health.

5. Require a detailed explanation of the role that local health departments will play in providing mental health, alcohol and drug services. They are supposed to soon begin assessing people with alcohol and drug problems and then refer them on for treatment. I believe assessment and treatment should be at one location as the more hoops these people have to jump through to get help the less likely they will follow through. In the past, these services were usually combined at the local mental health clinic. We all need to know exactly how the local health departments will be used. We don't need more confusion.

6. Obtain a detailed financial disclosure of mental health, alcohol and drug funding as it relates to the overall Department of Health budget.

7. Increasingly, members of the Alliance for the Mentally Ill and mental health centers are hearing, and law enforcement leaders are reporting, that the numbers of the mentally ill are dramatically increasing in jails. Recently, Davidson County Sheriff Gayle Ray reported a 100% increase over the past year. The Department of Health should initiate a statewide study to see if this is so, why it is happening and how these people are being treated in jail. If these reports are true,

"It's not fair. Jail is not the place a mentally ill person to get better." Sheriff Ray

recommendations should be made by the Department of Health for preventing the use of jails for mentally ill people who have not committed crimes.

8. In 1992 the legislature passed a bill for the sale or lease of unused mental health institute property to provide funding "for the specific purposes of planning and construction of mental health facilities, as well as for the transition of patients from an institutional setting into community programs." I understand that since this bill was passed a sizeable section of Lakeshore Mental Health Institute property was given to Knoxville for a park. If so, why was it allowed when funding is so badly needed for community housing and that land is so valuable? I recommend that the Department of Health prepare a proposal for the use of unused lands to provide funding for badly needed housing for the mentally ill. (See Acts 1992, ch 898, 12-2-117, Public Property, Printing and Contracts pa. 386-87).

9. If the bill for merger moves forward, support Senator Roscoe Dixon's amendment for the establishment of an "outside watchdog" ombudsmen, such as the Attorney General's office.

10. If the bill moves forward, support Senator Roscoe Dixon's amendment that each Bureau in the Department of Health be headed by an Assistant Commissioner.

And last, aside from the above which directly relates to the proposed merger, I want to use this opportunity to ask for your support for two bills which will be of great benefit to people with mental illness and severe emotional problems:

- SB2798, Senator Rochelle's bill that provides for mental health insurance parity.
- SB2532, Senator ~~Rochelle~~'s bill that provides for mental health "safety net" services.

End with quote from this mornings Tennessean editorial

Thank you.

10A • Wednesday, February 18/ 1998 — THE TENNESSEAN

EDITORIALS

Little surprise on BHO

TENNESSEAN 2-18-98

TennCare Partners needs radical attention

FOR $350 million a year, Tennessee's two behavioral health organizations can certainly work better than the evidence to date.

And when their clients happen to be the least powerful, the state simply shouldn't tolerate failure.

The latest blow to TennCare Partners, the state's health insurance program covering mental illness, came in an audit report of one of the two companies, Tennessee Behavioral Health, last week. TBH and Premier Behavioral Systems receive $350 million a year to provide mental health and substance abuse services to TennCare recipients.

The state Comptroller's Office concluded that TBH owed $20 million to providers and hospitals. Looking at a sample 277 claims, auditors cited TBH for wrongly denying benefits to nearly a third of the claims in its review.

The report went on to say that benefits often were paid off late if at all. By not paying providers properly, the company violates its contract with the state, according to the audit.

Obviously, such a circumstance adds to the troubles of patients seeking help. But the failure to pay providers hurts the very people who can help those in need.

TBH blamed the state's system of billing for at least part of the problem, but officials also said they were working with the state to correct the problems even before the report came out.

State officials have stopped any additional money for TennCare Partners until progress is made. A consultant has been hired to oversee claims and management at the companies. But the state will be lucky to get out of this without paying even more. It's having to refile some 25,000 claims.

The legislature should simply say "enough." For more than a year now, lawmakers have heard just how bad things were in TennCare Partners. What used to be dismissed as "anecdotal" evidence has become indisputable: The system isn't working.

An independent review of the Partners program, completed in September and October last year and only recently released, showed that care was haphazard at best. Partners offered no prevention program and little follow-up. Case management was used sparingly if at all for many patients. Those turned down for help weren't told why, according to the reports, and often had no recourse to an appeal of the decision.

The system isn't working for patients. It's not working for providers. And it's certainly not working for this state.

The issue of merging the Department of Mental Health and Mental Retardation has become secondary. Indeed, the legislature seems reluctant to make the move.

But radical attention to TennCare Partners can't wait. Legislators must insist on changes. They should require penalties if necessary to force the companies to comply. And they should act quickly.

Tennessee is paying a big price for TennCare Partners. But that's nothing compared to those who are suffering and can't get help. They need the legislature's immediate attention. ■

G-1 37212

TENNESSEAN 6-24-98

TennCare Partners reform is right

To the Editor:

Winston Churchill said of politics: "It would be a great reform in politics if wisdom could be made to spread as easily and as rapidly as folly." Gov. Don Sundquist's announced intent to reform TennCare Partners, the state's mental health-care program for the poor and uninsured, shows that wisdom is spreading in the reformation of public policy.

From its implementation in July 1996, it seemed TennCare Partners was doomed to failure. Deep program cuts indicated thousands of Tennesseans were not getting the proper care and treatment they so desperately needed to fight the debilitating effects of mental illness.

The behavioral health organizations (BHOs) set up to administer TennCare Partners were slow to process claims, which placed many providers in financial limbo. Pharmacy benefits, so critical in the care of mental illness, were poorly managed.

What's more, TennCare Partners recipients had to prove — in two failed trials — that older, less potent medications to manage mental illness were not working before being allowed to take newer and more effective medications. This requirement placed a tremendous burden of proof on consumers.

Sundquist deserves praise for the recent steps he's taken to improve TennCare Partners. The governor's announced intention to rewrite the mental health and mental retardation code elevates his commitment, beyond that of a quick fix, in response to public criticism and shows a genuine concern for improving the lives of the mentally ill.

George Spain
1101 Sixth Ave. N. 37208

THE TENNESSEAN

6B • Wednesday, July 29/ 1998 — THE TENNESSEAN

LOCAL NEWS

Three to help rewrite state mental health law

By DUREN CHEEK
Staff Writer

HEALTH

Three Nashvillians — Elise McMillan, Carol Westlake, and George Spain — were among 10 persons appointed by Gov. Don Sundquist yesterday to a commission that will work on a proposed rewrite of state laws regarding mental health and mental retardation.

The group's work would be presented to the state legislature for review.

McMillan, the parent of a child with Down syndrome, is director of development for the John F. Kennedy Center and statewide senior vice president of the Tennessee Association of Retarded Citizens (ARC).

Westlake is executive director of the Tennessee Disability Coalition, a coalition of about 30 groups who deal with disability issues.

Spain is chief executive officer of Centerstone Mental Health Center, Inc.

"Each of these appointees bring to the group a different perspective on mental health, mental retardation and disability issues in Tennessee," Sundquist said in a written statement.

A rewrite of the mental health and mental retardation code is one of a series of steps the governor announced back in March that he was going to take to address problems with mental health and mental retardation services provided by the state.

"It's outdated and needs to be updated relative to what's happening in today's society," Beth Fortune, the governor's spokeswoman, said.

Laws dealing with mental retardation were written back when most mental retardation services were provided in institutions. Today, there is more emphasis on community placement with "many thousand" people being treated in communities, she said.

Also, mental health laws were written before the advent of managed health care and also need to be updated, Fortune said.

The commission is expected to complete its task in about 18 months.

Other members of the commission are:

- Gaylon Booker of Memphis, senior vice president for the National Cotton Council and parent of a son with disabilities.
- Lee Chase, executive director of a regional rehabilitation center in Johnson City.
- Carolyn Cowans of Memphis, president of Arlington Development Center Parents.
- Andy Fox, former executive director of the Southeast Mental health Center in Memphis.
- Anne Ince of Knoxville, a member of the national Mental Health Association Board.
- Harold North, a Chattanooga attorney and president-elect of Big Brothers/Big Sisters of Chattanooga.
- June Palmer of Dyersburg, state president of the Tennessee Alliance for the Mentally Ill, Inc.

Four state lawmakers will also serve on the commission: Sens. Roy Herron of Dresden and Curtis Person of Memphis and Reps. Mary Ann Eckles of Murfreesboro and Page Walley of Toone, in rural West Tennessee. ■

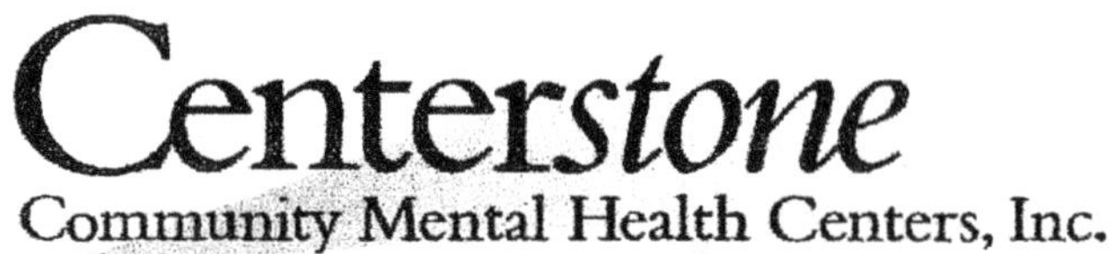

What is Centerstone Community Mental Health Centers, Inc.?

- 501(c)(3) not-for-profit organization
- Common parent company supporting its membership of providers – legally a "sole member". Parent company for:
    - Columbia Area Mental Health Center
    - Dede Wallace Center
    - Harriett Cohn Center
    - Highland Rim Mental Health Center
    - Luton Mental Health Services
- Not a "merger", "holding company", nor provider
- Authority to contract for its members though members may still contract individually if necessary.
- Provides overall governance for its members. Single policies, procedures, and monitoring of financial affairs.
- The "supported organizations" retain their identity (local name) and rights to ownership.
- Risks are shared and incentives aligned to promote coordinated efforts.

Centerstone Community Mental Health Centers, Inc.

Creation

- December 1, 1997, Centerstone, a 501(c)(3) non-profit corporation, formed a "parent company" for four affiliates:

  Columbia Area Mental Health Center
  Dede Wallace Center
  Harriett Cohn Center
  Highland Rim Mental Health Center

- July 1, 1998, Luton Mental Health Services joined the Centerstone affiliation.
- January 1, 1999, Centerstone began the management of Elam Mental Health Clinic.
- July, 2000 Centerstone's five affiliates fully merged.

Facts

- The largest behavioral health provider in Tennessee and one of the largest in the nation.
- Serves nearly 40,000 individuals and families annually: 56% adults; 44% children and youth
- 1100+ employees
- 23 volunteer board members
- 56 sites located in 26 Middle Tennessee counties
- $51,000,000 revenue:
  - 66% TennCare
  - 27% Government Contracts
  - 3%% Client Fees and Insurance
  - 2% Other
  - 2% Fund Raising

New Initiatives

- Research
- Elder services
- Telemedicine
- Primary Care Integration
- Crisis Management Strategies Critical Incident Stress Management Program
- Fully integrated internet-based clinical record technology
- Integration of academic services for child and adolescent residential and day treatment programs.

Pending Initiatives

- Partnership with Memorial Hospital/Tennessee Christian Medical Center Gateway in Clarksville for operation of hospital-based emergency walk-in mental health clinic
- Restructure Nashville's Harbor House from long-term residential to transition and diversion for adult acute care consumers
- Collaborating with state and community health and social agencies to organize services for refugees and immigrants.
- Partnership with Middle Tennessee Mental Health Institute to create inpatient services program for Centerstone consumers, staffed with Centerstone psychiatrist
- Partnership with Nashville Consortium of Safety Net Providers to expand primary care, behavioral and dental health services to Davidson County's uninsured.

Size and Location

- Facilities in 20 mid-Tennessee counties. Services to 26 counties. Largest behavioral health provider in Middle Tennessee. Corporate offices in Nashville.
- 900 employees
- $33,000,000 budget
- 25 percent of entire TennCare population
- 27 member governing board, with representatives for each of its five centers
- 21 member Board of Trustees, composed of county executives and metro council persons
- Four Development Boards, for local fundraising
- Consumer and Family Advocacy Council composed of Middle Tennessee consumer and family leaders

Why Did We Do It?

- Respond to the requirements of managed care.
- Assure the continuance of volunteer, community controlled services.
- Improve and expand services throughout Middle Tennessee. Cross-fertilization of best practices.
- Gain geographical presence, market share, strength, and influence. Oneness creates power.
- Streamline organizations, improve efficiency and effectiveness.
- Create larger pool of talent and resources to draw from.
- Enhance quality, continuity of care, and financial performance.
- Increase employee opportunities and security.
- Strengthen negotiating and contracting abilities.
- Coordinate efforts in developing new alliances, affiliations, and networks to assure integrated delivery of services.

How Was It Done?

- Pinnacle Health (Columbia Area, Harriett Cohn, Highland Rim) formed in February, 1997.
- Centerstone (Pinnacle and Dede Wallace Center) formed December 1, 1997.
- Centerstone and Luton affiliate July 1, 1998.
- Initial meetings and agreements by the two directors.
- Formal approval to negotiate by boards and formation of Ad Hoc negotiation committees.
- Selection of consultant and attorneys. Sign letter of intent and confidentiality agreement.
- Determination of organization structure, make up of management staff, placement of key staff and board composition.
- Due diligence study conducted.
- Determined internal and external communication process; periodic updates to staff.
- New charter, by-laws, employment agreements of top executives approved by Ad Hoc negotiating committee.
- Selected name i.e. Centerstone (Federal Trademark)
- Management staff begins detailed discussions and decisions on personnel policies, liability and health insurance, etc. Staff integration plans developed, job descriptions, organizational table finalized. Transition business plan developed.
- Boards ratify Ad Hoc Committee motions, elect representatives for governing board for the new parent company – Centerstone. Boards of Pinnacle and Dede Wallace Center and Luton vote themselves out of existence.

- Final signatures to all legal documents. All facilities now licensed as Centerstone. News releases.

- Centerstone Community Mental Health Centers, Inc. board meets and passes initial operational motions ratifying actions by original member boards. Budget integrated and approved. Centerstone is now a reality!

- Management staff retreat held. Integration, integration, integration! Full integration may take 2-3 years.

- Prepare for negatives, staff confusion and opposition, some good staff will likely resign. Importance of executive and management staff working closely together – keep eyes focused on basis for the affiliation, the positive potential.

- Integration of financial costs offset by savings in insurance and purchasing power.

- New affiliation opportunities begin occurring.

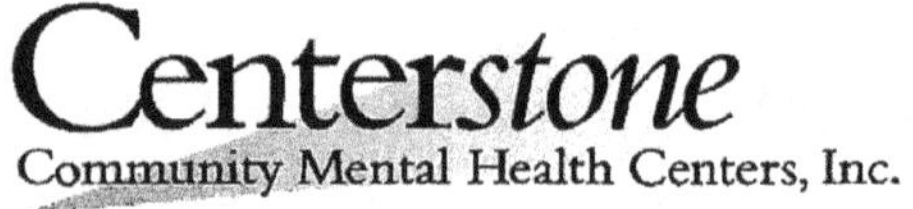

Centerstone Community Mental Health Centers, Inc.

The Future of Mental Health in the New Millennium

We stand upon the threshold of great changes and improvements in mental health care. These challenges will come from new research discoveries, changes in services and funding expectations and major health and social problems of our youth and elderly.

Research is increasingly leading to the possibility that brain disorders such as schizophrenia and bi-polar illnesses will be prevented by genetic treatment.

Advances in medication research are steadily producing highly effective medicines with limited side effects. We near the time when curing these illnesses will be achieved.

Increasingly, medical schools will turn out primary care doctors, internists, family practitioners, and pediatricians who know how to treat major psychiatric illnesses. In time, this will improve care, reduce costs, and help diminish stigma and prejudice.

Primary care physicians and their assistants will increasingly use specially designed diagnostic tools, including computerized telephone services, to diagnose and treat mental illnesses in their own offices or they will include behavioral specialists within their practice.

Purchasers of services will seek providers who offer fully integrated systems of primary and behavioral health care. Competition will continue to increase.

Consumer and family education on mental illness, symptoms, treatment and best practice providers will become a part of the internet and will positively influence the seeking of early treatment, choices in the best providers and compliance with treatment.

Telecommunications will be available to emergency rooms and primary care practices for specialty evaluations and consultations.

The use of hospitals for treatment will continue to decline while the demand for home health and community-based treatment will continue to increase.

By 2050, almost 18.5% of the population will be over age 85 with an accompanying marked increase demand for specialized geriatric services.

Childhood and adolescent violence, alcohol and drug abuse, academic failures and other major youth problems will, for the foreseeable future, continue. The State and community will seek preventive programs for pre-school and early grades.

~ ~ ~ ~ ~ ~ ~ ~ ~ ~ ~ ~ ~ ~ ~

So, how should these influences shape Centerstone's future? What should Centerstone become? What will we look like?

We will help bring the treatment of mental illness into the mainstream of medical. Our services will be integrated with primary care practices and county health departments by the combining of staffs, locations, and by formal affiliations.

We will form strong partnerships with major educational/medical institutions thereby contributing to research, education, the provision of highly specialized services, the design of new technologies, and the development of health insurance for which we will be a primary provider.

We will, through expansion of our own services and by integrating with others, become a leading provider of care for the elderly.

In collaboration with other systems, we will make our communities better and stronger by developing extensive preventive services for high-risk pre-school and early grade children.

Centerstone will create an institution with the will, the qualities and the image of leadership.

Reduction in Hospitalization – A Priority

As we gear up for risk contracting it is essential that we are prepared with a commitment and a plan to maximize the responsible use of all our services to reduce hospital admissions and length of stay. All of Centerstone staff and services that can influence these reductions must be committed to this priority.

I believe our goal should be to responsibly lead Tennessee with the lowest rate of hospitalization and when that is consistently achieved the goal then shifts to the nation. We see how the experience of doing battle has unified our staff. Esprit de corps can result from striving toward and ultimately achieving a quality in our services that is so strong and so well run that we become the "best" in caring for people in the community.

First, we need the total commitment of our management staff to begin now in making full use of the services we have to prevent hospitalization.

Second, we need a plan which is constructed from ideas and recommendations from mobile crisis, case management, medical staff, hospital liaison, outpatient therapists, residential managers, drop-in center directors, etc. They need to tell us ways to improve what we are already doing and what needs to be added to reduce hospitalization. They need to share in an on-going improvement process. They need to receive the monthly hospital reports which Brad will provide.

Third, a monthly report should be prepared which provides:

- Admission rates per thousand members broken down by:
  - County of residence
  - Adult/Child
  - Mobile crisis service area
  - Both mental health and dual diagnosis
  - First admission/recidivism
  - If already in our system, what services were being provided
  - Where hospitalized
- On-going comparisons showing by numbers and graph:
  - Last year (by County, area, total)
  - State rates
  - Non-Centerstone areas that are running lower
- Adverse incident and complaint report to see if there are increases related to reducing hospitalization

While more may be added to the reports, they should be as clear and simple as possible. The reports should be provided monthly to all the key managers and reviewed at all clinical operations and management meetings to assure that on-going attention occurs and that ideas for improvements are constantly obtained.

Other Comments:

- Don't worry about how we compare to the nation until we are consistently the best in Tennessee. Don't delay getting started until every needed resource is available – use what we have, shift its focus if necessary and get on with it.
- As we begin seeing a trend of improvement, recognize those who are making it happen and tell the board about them.
- Don't forget the consumers, have them involved in creating the plan and keep them involved. They will help.
- A small, on-going task force should be assigned to assure the plan is being followed or changed if it isn't working.
- Measurable goals should be considered, i.e., rates per admission/hospital days
- If we believe that good continuity of care can reduce recidivism, then we should seek to have our own hospital unit for Centerstone's consumers. Bob and I have had an initial talk with MTMHI. If Joe Carobene and the state are willing to consider this, we should make this one of the plan's priorities.
- The development of a telemental health hub site at MTMHI or another hospital should be considered in the plan.

George Spain
May 7, 2001

Mental And Physical Ca

BY SHARON H. FITZGERALD

Most parents have experienced this: Their child doesn't want to go to school and feigns a tummy ache. But then the child vomits, and what was simple fear has escalated into physical illness.

"There's a well-known history with children at the beginning of the school year who have anxiety related to separation. They may start throwing up and even get temperatures. Terror can cause physical symptoms, as can anxiety related to moving from the familiar to the unfamiliar," says George Spain, chief executive officer of Centerstone Community Mental Health Centers, a Nashville-based nonprofit organization providing community mental health services through six Middle Tennessee centers.

Alleviating such anxiety for children is just one of many reasons why Centerstone's Tullahoma facility, Highland Rim Mental Health Center, teamed up with the locally owned, private Pediatric Clinic in Tullahoma. Today, a Centerstone employee, Nancy Garrison, works at the Pediatric Clinic. Garrison is a registered nurse with a doctorate in psychology, and it's her job to treat the mental and behavioral problems of the Pediatric Clinic's young patients *at the clinic*, rather than requiring families to seek that help at another location.

"She's our employee, but she goes to work there every day, has an office there and provides counseling to the children and the parents and does evaluations," Spain explains. "If the pediatrician decides that a child's problem may be a mental health or behavioral problem, the pediatrician goes right down the hallway and gets Nancy, brings her right in and introduces her to the parents and child."

This pilot program was launched about a year ago, but the idea was two years in the making. "And it was preceded by a good working relationship that existed with this private group of pediatricians," Spain adds. The Pediatric Clinic even handles the billing of Garrison's services for Highland Rim.

While convenience for families is one positive aspect of the program, there's much more. "Yes, it's convenient, but also there's certainly less stigma with treatment right there in the Pediatric Clinic," Spain explains. "With many people who are referred from pediatricians and family practitioners, they simply never make it over to the mental health center. They may be referred and they may have an appointment, but for many reasons, perhaps anxiety, they just don't follow through. In this case, you

...re Under One Roof

have immediate access to them in an environment which they are familiar with and most likely have a good bit of trust built around."

More integration of mental and behavioral treatment with primary care is a goal for Centerstone, says Spain.

"I'm working on expanding this," he says. "This is an area that our board has made a commitment to, to find every way we can to integrate with primary care. So many of the people we serve have other medical problems and sometimes have difficulty accessing those problems. The more we can integrate, the better it will be for them. Many people see internists, family practitioners and pediatricians when depression and anxiety may well be underlying the symptoms they are showing. The more we can integrate with them, the more comfortable the patients can be and the more services we can get to them."

Centerstone has placed a staff member in Centerville's new public health department facility, and plans are in place to put a Centerstone employee in Ashland City when Cheatham County's new public health clinic opens. These mental health professionals in public healthcare settings will serve adults and children.

Spain says, with the advent of better psychotropic medications, more and more internists, family practitioners and pediatricians are treating mental and behavioral problems — and recognizing the connections between mental and physical health.

"That's improved tremendously," he says. "I envision the day when there will be a shift to primary care doctors caring for more and more people with mental illness. Again, that's a reason for our being involved with them."

Yet, Spain adds, "Even with all the enlightenment of our age, I still am aware that for many people, making that first appointment and walking through the doors of the mental health center are very, very difficult things. That explains the reason there are a lot of failures in keeping appointments and following through." The result can be an escalation of symptoms and even eventual hospitalization or emergency-room treatment, he adds.

That's why integrated programs such as the Tullahoma project can make such a difference, Spain says. And he points to a "wonderfully integrated program" in Morristown that offers primary care, dental care, alcohol and drug care, and mental health services all under one roof.

"That's what my vision is," he says, "to create in the area we serve."

Minority and Immigrant Populations - Special Service Needs

This report is in response to the Centerstone 2001-2002 Strategic Plan's objective: "Provide report to the Board describing special service needs for minority/immigrant populations living in Centerstone's service area by July 1, 2002." In this report the term minority is limited to race and ethnicity.

-- George Spain

> "America draws strength from its cultural diversity. The contributions of racial and ethnic minorities have suffused all areas of contemporary life. Diversity has made our nation a more vibrant and open society, ablaze in ideas, perspectives, and innovations. But the full potential of our diverse, multicultural society cannot be realized until all Americans, including racial and ethnic minorities, gain access to quality health care that meets their needs."
>
> Dr. David Satcher, Surgeon General, 2001

Middle Tennessee's Racial Composition

Nashville has received a great honor and with it a great responsibility. Nashville is now recognized as one of the nation's "new Ellis Islands." Among the 100 largest metropolitan areas, Nashville had the greatest ratio of new legal immigrants arriving in 1991-1998 compared with the foreign-born population living here in 1990. Nashville's ratio was double the nation's average.

According to a recent Metro Government report, one out of every six Nashvillians was born outside the United States. A Metro school report states that four thousand five hundred (4,500) immigrant children are enrolled as English Language Learners. The National Center for Immigration Studies predicts that "absent any change in U.S. immigration policy, the immigrant population in Nashville will almost certainly grow in the decades to come."

Of Davidson County's 570,000 people, 147,000 are African American and 85,000 are of other races, the largest number of these being Latinos. Two out of five Nashvillians are non-white. It should be anticipated that in not many years the combined minority populations in Nashville will exceed that of whites. This projection is also anticipated for all the United States by 2050.

In the other twenty-five counties served by Centerstone, there are nearly 1.2 million people of whom 90% are white, 8% African American, and 2% Latino. In one county, Bedford, Hispanics are almost 8% of the population. When these counties are combined with Davidson County, 14% of the 1.8 million population are African American and 3% Latino.

Nationally, Latinos now exceed African Americans. By 2050, it is projected that one of four Americans will be Latino. In the past ten years, their numbers have grown to at least 57,000 in middle Tennessee, a 345% increase.

Culture, Race, and Ethnicity – A 2002 Supplement to Mental Health: Findings of the Surgeon General

- Mental illnesses are real, disabling conditions affecting all populations, regardless of race or ethnicity.
- Striking disparities in mental health care are found for racial and ethnic minorities:
    - Minorities have less access to and availability of services.
    - Minorities are less likely to receive needed services.
    - Minorities in treatment often receive poorer quality care.
    - Minorities are underrepresented in mental health research.
- Disparities impose a greater disability burden on minorities.
- Racism and discrimination are stressful events that adversely affect health and mental health.
- Mistrust of mental health services is an important reason deterring minorities from seeking treatment.
- The cultures of racial and ethnic minorities alter the types of mental health services they need.

- Errors in diagnosis are made more often in African Americans than for whites.
- About 40 percent of Latino Americans in the 1990 Census reported they do not speak English well. Very few mental health providers are Spanish speaking.

Surgeon General's Vision for the Future

- Continue to expand the science base regarding racial and ethnic minority mental health.
- Increase access to treatment through geographical availability, integration with primary care, and improved language access. Increase care to incarcerated, homeless, and children living in out-of-home placements.
- Reduce barriers to care by overcoming stigma, increasing mental health insurance parity.
- Improve quality of services using evidenced-based professional treatment guidelines and research.
- Support capacity development by expanding minority representation among providers, administrators, policy makers, researchers, etc.
- Promote mental health by building on intrinsic community strengths, ethnic values, spirituality, and strategies that strengthens families.

Centerstone's Status

- Centerstone is in compliance with Title VI – the federal law that deals with nondiscrimination in federally assisted programs. (See Appendix A for Policies and Procedures).
- In November 2001, Centerstone had almost 24,000 active consumers, 20,959 reporting their race as:

White	16,335	78%
African Americans	4,057	19.4%
Latinos	326	1.5%
Other	241	1.1%

- A quick survey of staff showed that only 21 spoke a second language. Of these, four spoke Spanish.

- Of the 14 senior managers, two are of a minority race – African American and Latino.
- Of the 24 board members, three are of a minority race – African Americans.
- Formal cultural competency training is limited to a brief presentation during orientation of new employees.
- Present use of interpreters include a telephonic interpretation service, an interpreter in Bedford County, as well as use of family and friends (see Appendix B for Case Example).
- While Centerstone has several cultural competency policies, they are limited. We have not comprehensive policies or plan.
- Executive Management are active participants in:
  - Tennessee Mental Health Planning Council's Cultural Competence Committee
  - Nashville Task Force on Refugees and Immigrants
  - Encuentro Latino Mental Health
  - Middle Tennessee Coalition of Health Care Providers (Coalition is surveying mid-Tennessee mental health providers regarding Latino services)
  - Involved in collaborative efforts with other providers for Robert Wood Johnson Foundation grant to improve communication with Latinos.

Special Service Needs in Centerstone's Service Area

- A culturally competent system of care which holds diverse cultures in high esteem, doing everything possible to ensure access to care, regardless of difference in language, cultural background or social status.
- Access to specially trained interpreters and/or bilingual and bicultural providers who are well trained and experienced in cultural competency.
- Diagnostic protocols which include assessment of cultural influences.
- Marketing strategies designed specifically for ethnically diverse populations.
- Policies, procedures, continuing education and research which ensure that services are accessible, appropriate, and acceptable to diverse populations.

- Inclusion of ethnic diversity on boards and management.
- Bilingual forms, information materials, etc.

Recommendations

- The Board should commit Centerstone to becoming a national leader in providing culturally competent services to immigrants, refugees, and minorities.
- Comprehensive cultural competency policies and plan should be developed by management and approved by Board. Minority representatives should assist.
- Amending mission/vision statements to include Centerstone's responsibility to minorities (See Meharry example Appendix C).
- Fill one board position with a Latino leader.
- As management positions come open, minority representation should be given special attention.
- Board, management, and staff take cultural competency training.
- Diagnostic protocols should include cultural assessment (see example Appendix D).
- Marketing plan should be developed for all minorities including written materials, advertising, etc.
- Seek grants that will help improve minority services.
- Establish plan for building language communication with trained interpreters and actively seek bilingual/bicultural clinicians. Consider uses of telemedicine.
- Develop ongoing cultural education plan for entire organization to assure that staff understand policies and carry them out.
- Senior management assume responsibility for maintaining collaborative relationships with immigrant, refugee, and minority organizations.
- Establish ongoing self evaluation to determine effectiveness of policies and procedures on access, appropriateness and acceptableness of services for immigrants and minorities. Make an annual progress report to Board.

- Develop national research regarding effectiveness of treatment of minority populations. Seek grants.
- Title VI compliance must be maintained.

> "Racial and ethnic minorities collectively experience a high disability burden from unmet mental health needs. Despite the progress in understanding the causes of mental illness and the tremendous advances in finding effective mental health treatments, far less is known about the mental health of African Americans, American Indians, and Alaska Natives, Asian Americans, and Pacific Islanders, and Hispanic Americans.
> "The Nation has far to go to eliminate racial and ethnic disparities in mental health. Mental health as a whole will be enhanced substantially by improving the health of racial and ethnic minorities."
>
> Dr. David Satcher, Surgeon General, 2001
> (See Appendix E)

In conclusion, see Appendix F for questions related to your own origins and culture.

> "Remember, we are all children of immigrants."
> George Spain, 2002

Memorandum regarding establishing a cooperative relationship for developing crisis intervention programs among ***The Centerstone, USA ; Department of Psychology, The Sci-Tech University and Seventh hospital of HangZhou , China***

Crisis intervention programs now recommended as the important and effective method for dealing with crises and disaster in all over the world. They have been shown to be effective for promoting effective crisis response capability of all potential clients. There is growing need in China. For the purpose of updating the knowledge of clinical applications of crisis intervention, thereby, enhancing the quality of education&training in China, ***The Centerstone , American; Department of Psychology, The Sci-Tech University and The Seventh Hospital Of HangZhou*** agree to establish a cooperative relationship.

This agreement includes:

The Centerstone,USA will provide Chinese behavioral healthcare professionals with systematic training courses and will support ***Department of Psychology, The Sci-Tech University and The Seventh Hospital Of HangZhou*** to establish the same services in ZheJiang Province , China and carry out correlative clinical education&training projects.

The Centerstone,USA will participate in designing and monitoring the all training program and provide the necessary education materials in English for ***Department of Psychology, The Sci-Tech University*** to translate and use in its program. At the same time, ***Department of Psychology, The Sci-Tech University, ZheJiang*** will be responsible for monitor and evaluation of quality of all programs.

The Seventh Hospital Of HangZhou will responsible for implementing all detailed practice of education& training programs, and provide all local expenses and domestic traveling fees for the trainer(s). A training honorarium will be paid to ***The Centerstone,USA*** and ***Department of Psychology, The Sci-Tech University*** to cover other costs and for their efforts.

The Centerstone,USA will accept 2-3 professionals of ***Department of Psychology, The Sci-Tech University and The Seventh Hospital Of HangZhou*** to learn program management and being the trainer in the American. ***The Centerstone,USA*** also can help the cooperant partner to make contact with the local behavioral healthcare services in USA to visit. Partial expenses for Chinese professionals while in USA will be their own responsibility.

This agreement is only an informal agreement to evidence the establishment of the project and the formal agreement and the detailed information will be discussed in the early period of 2006.

Helena Guo

A deputy to the Centerstone Company

Tennessee, USA

Signature:________________________

Date:_______/_________ /_________

Ge, Lie Zhong

Head & executive director

Department of Psychology, the Sci-Tech University

ZheJiang Province, China

Signature:________________________

Date:_______/_________ /_________

Zhao, Guo Qiu

Director of the Hospital

The Seventh Hospital Of HangZhou

ZheJiang Province, China

Signature:________________________

Date:_______/_________ /_________

Centerstone Partnership with China –2005

China Background

- Crisis management is becoming one of major focus for government and public.
- The social structure changes create significant change in work environment and family structure. Once stable work and family life and structure are largely diminished due to economic growth.
- Chinese people become more and more isolated with increasing stress.
- More and more people realize their unmet emotional and psychological needs.
- Mental health is just wakening in China, infrastructure is under developed with very limited providers.
- China is becoming more and more focused on developing community healthcare system.
- Developing a mental health system in established community healthcare center will be model or trend in near future.
- Established physical structures are already in place.
- Basic clinical counseling structure is already established recently.
- Strong support from Government
- There are monetary resources to support and develop the projects.

How Centerstone Could Benefit from the Collaboration?

- Introducing Centerstone to China.
- Helping China set up cutting edge community health center
- Centerstone mainly providing software to a established hardware system, so it cost effective
- Helping Centerstone set track records on providing mental health consultant services to mental or physical health services centers.
- Helping Centerstone to establish a comprehensive community health services model
- Centerstone could establish national and international partner chain services system, In that each partner will contribute certain or fix amount annual profit to Centerstone.
- The established procedure and system can be used as product to be purchased by other community health centers in China.
- Centerstone will own at least half of the completed product (Chinese version of the system).

The Important Fact

China is growing very rapidly. They have much broader contact with outside of the world than before. They will have this comprehensive system established with our help or with someone else's help. My hope is that Centerstone is the one.

The roles of each participant:

Organization	Roles and Contribution
Centerstone - Zhao, Guoqiu	Phase I • Providing crisis management Information Resources • Providing experiences in managing and practicing in mental health field • Reputation of Centerstone • Assisting China partner to set up the program Phase II • Advice and guidance for their clinical practice • Assisting to establish clinical programs in community health centers • Assisting to set up clinical procedures and management system • Assisting to set up data Recording and management system
Zhejiang Science and Technology University	• Critical incident stress management foundation center • Coordinating resources between U.S and China • Translating information and training material into Chinese • Localizing or customerlizing the information into Chinese culture • Follow up research on critical incident stress interventions • Teaching and training critical incident responding Team
Zhejiang Mental health Association Hangzhou Mental health Hospital Community Health Center Zhao, Guoqiu Wang, Yiqiang Liao, Hong	• Recruiting trainees • Organizing training courses • Coordinating Services and interventions • Establish network critical incident responding Team • Providing mental health services • Outreach and education • Providing crisis intervention services in safe and more culturally acceptable environment

Department of Health director

Ni, Rong

This was not successful

SS. - 2018